# TOTAL
# ABS

# ACKNOWLEDGMENTS

This publication is based on articles written by **Mike Carlson; Alwyn Cosgrove; Jon Finkel; Rob Fitzgerald; Bill Geiger; Alan Gurler; Myatt Murphy; Jimmy Pena; Jim Stoppani, Ph.D.; Eric Velazquez;** and **Joe Wuebben**

Cover photography by **Marc Royce**

Photography and illustrations by **Dylan Coulter, Michael Darter, Ian Logan, Robert Reiff, Marc Royce,** and **Pavel Ythjall**

Editor-in-Chief of *Muscle & Fitness* is **Shawn Perine**

Project editor is **Joe Wuebben**

Project creative director is **Anthony Scerri**

Project copy editor is **Cat Perry**

Project photo assistant is **Anthony Nolan**

Founding chairman is **Joe Weider.** Chairman and CEO of American Media, Inc., is **David Pecker.**

This book is available in quantity at special discounts for your group or organization. For further information, contact:

Triumph Books
814 North Franklin Street
Chicago, IL 60610
(800) 888-4741
fax (312) 280-5470
*www.triumphbooks.com*

ISBN: 978-1-60078-830-7

Printed in USA.

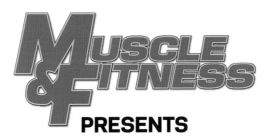

# MUSCLE & FITNESS PRESENTS

# TOTAL ABS

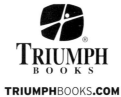

## TRIUMPH
### BOOKS

**TRIUMPH**BOOKS**.COM**

# CONTENTS

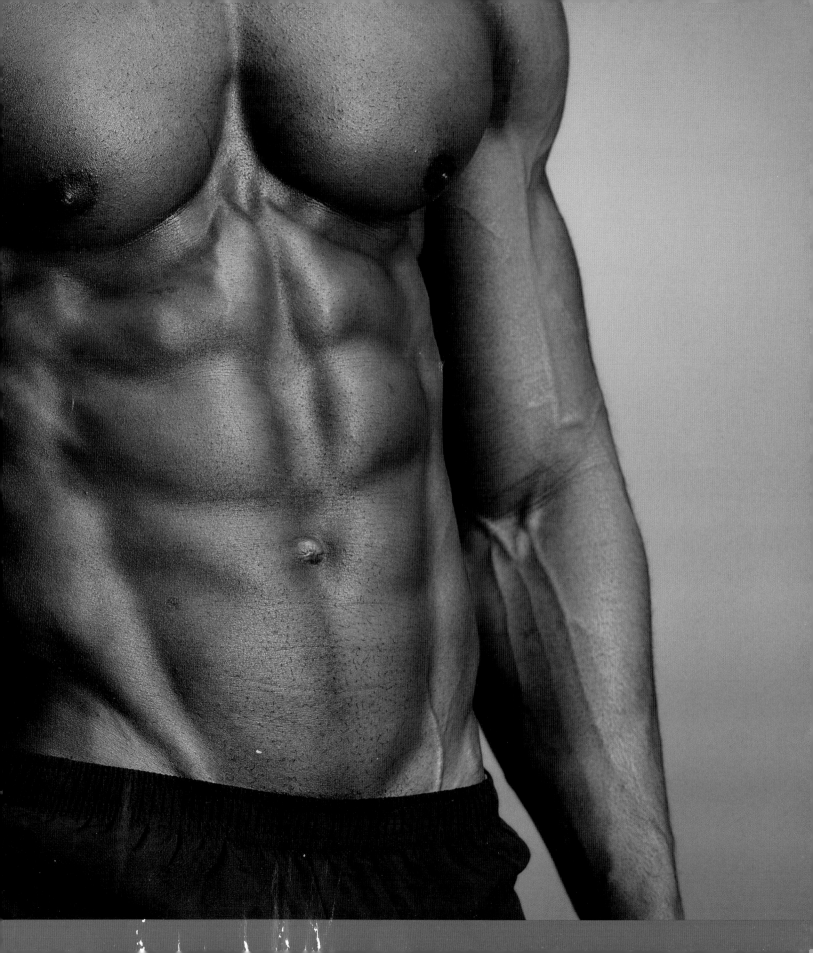

# FOREWORD

## SIX LITTLE BUMPS CAN MAKE A BIG DIFFERENCE

Two guys are walking down the beach (no, this isn't the start of a joke). After an intense workout, these training partners have decided to display the fruits of their labor down by the shore, where they make a friendly wager on whose physique will draw more admiring glances. One of the guys is big, with broad shoulders, a shadow-casting chest, and arms the size of legs. He also has a sizable midsection, with nary a hint of definition. The other isn't nearly as massive as his buddy, but has crisp conditioning, most noticeably in a six-pack so sharp you could strike a match on it. Which one of the two do you have winning the bet? If you're like me, you put your money on Mr. Abs.

The above scenario isn't entirely fictional; it's actually rooted in my own history. When I was 19 my training partner and I decided to make a cross-country pilgrimage from New York to bodybuilding's "mecca": Southern California. We'd both trained hard for the trip in an attempt to look like we belonged with the "in" crowd. At 5'9", I'd gotten myself up to 200 pounds for it—about 40 more than my birdlike bone structure was made to carry.

Feeling full of ourselves, we unpacked our luggage upon arriving at our hotel and then made a beeline to Muscle Beach in Venice. Wearing bathing suits and nothing else, we trained on the beach, making sure to keep our shoulders back and chests puffed out at all times.

Suddenly, in between sets of dips, a kid who was watching us train came up to me and asked, "Are you guys football players?"

"No, we're bodybuilders!" I quickly asserted, probably sounding more than a bit defensive. Actually, I was crestfallen. I'd worked so hard throughout my teens to be a bodybuilder, only to be mistaken for a…football player! (Keep in mind that in the '80s the NFL didn't have nearly as many physical specimens as it does today.)

When we returned to the hotel I took a sober look in the mirror. *Why didn't that kid ask me if I was a bodybuilder?* I wondered, as my eyes scanned my reflected image. I was big for sure, and proportioned, but I couldn't help notice the amorphous expanse between my chest and bathing suit. There was a faint shadow of three rows of abs there, but nothing to write home about. Truth is, I barely trained them. Then, when I estimated my body fat to be about 15%, the kid's comment began to make sense to me. And just like that, I got it. I understood how abdominals can make or break a physique.

The fact is that there's no muscle group with the same ability to impress. Maybe it's because they make up the most expansive part of the front of the body, while visually tying together the upper and lower halves. Or possibly because, since the time of the ancient Greeks, a well-developed midsection has signified health, strength, and vitality. Or it might have to do with the cultural perception forged by action stars like Bruce Lee, Sylvester Stallone, Arnold Schwarzenegger, and Jean-Claude Van Damme (you knew that Rocky was ready to kick ass and take names when his abdominals resembled the underside of an egg carton!).

Whatever your motivation, your decision to build a great set of abs will get you not only looking good, but healthy as well. How does having great abs equal good health? Well, to get them you have to put in some physical labor—exercises from a variety of angles—to work the rectus abdominis, the serratus, the obliques, and even the intercostals and serratus. In addition, you'll need to stick to a sound diet—one low in simple carbs and saturated fats. Add to that cardio—to help strip off any adipose tissue covering your efforts—and you're soon going to be feeling as good as you're looking.

This book has everything you need to develop your own set of *Muscle & Fitness* cover-worthy abs. You just add a little hard work. I won't lie to you, it takes effort and diligence to get great abs. But here's the good news: Once you start seeing results you'll be hooked on the process of getting them. The better they look, the more you'll want to work them.

Since my Muscle Beach incident, I decided to stop fighting my genetic lot, abandoning my quest to be massive. Instead, I set my sites on looking lean and proportioned. The goal became more Stallone than Schwarzenegger. These days I train my abs at the end of every workout, which means four to six times per week. I find it a good way to cool down and ease my way out of gym mode. Plus, to date, it's helped keep me from being mistaken for a 1980s football player again.

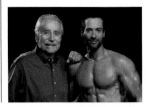

**More Power to You,**
## Shawn Perine
**Editor-in-Chief, *Muscle & Fitness***

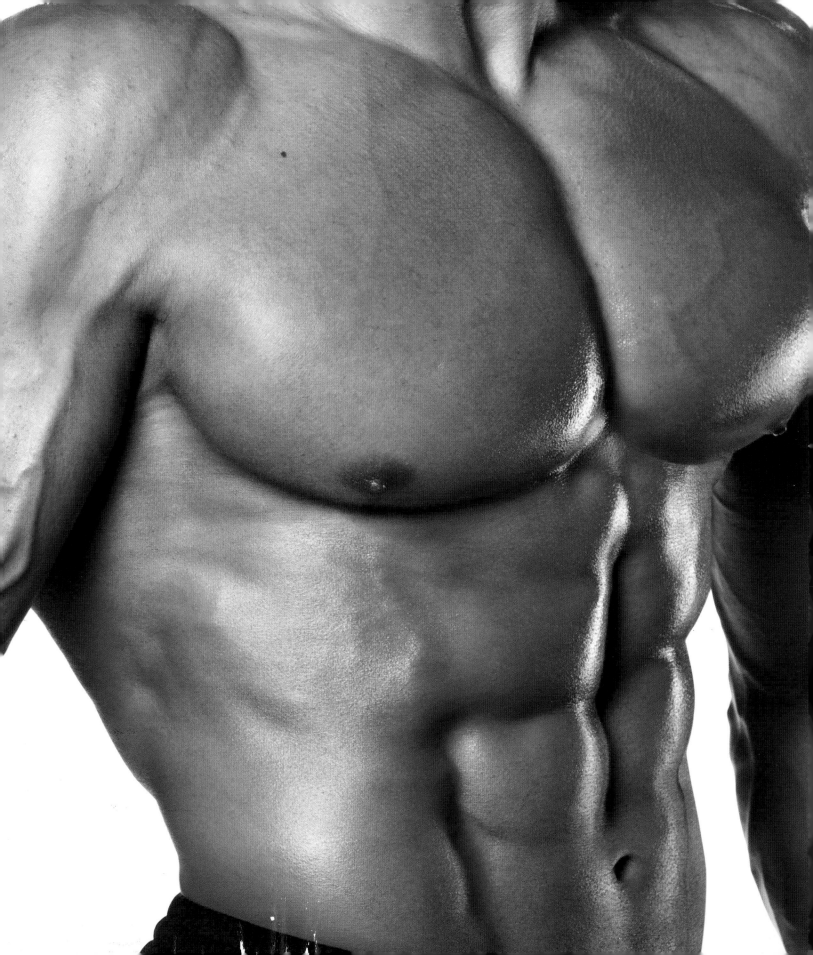

# AB TRAINING 101

**Is your pursuit of great abdominals all over the map? Take the guesswork out of finding your own defined six-pack with these simple guidelines.**

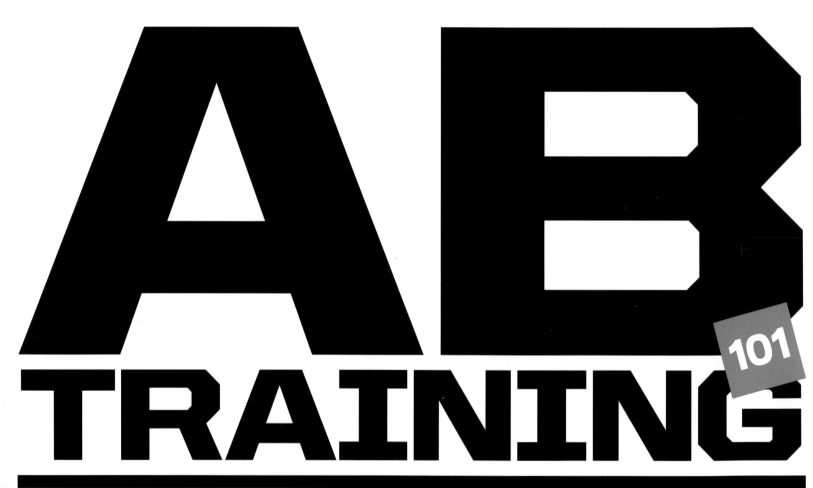

Pretend for a moment that your midsection is a map you're trying to navigate. You'd like to explore a number of different areas and regions, but you're not quite sure what's the best way to go about it. After all, when it comes to this terrain in particular, there are all sorts of conflicting opinions on how to navigate it most effectively and find the path to the ultimate six-pack. What you really need is the ab version of a high-tech GPS, something that will tell you how to arrive at your destination the quickest way possible. That's where *M&F* comes in. Think of this introductory chapter (and the rest of this book, for that matter) as your very own Abdominal Positioning System, telling you what areas to train, when to train them, and how—with no risk of making any wrong turns along the way.

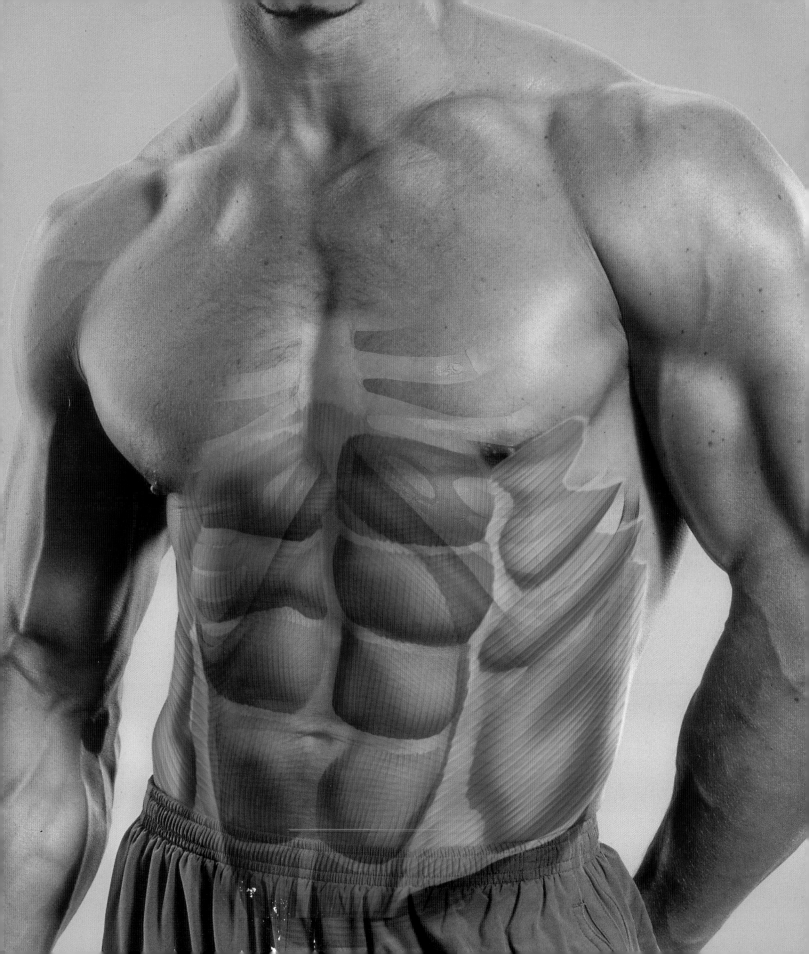

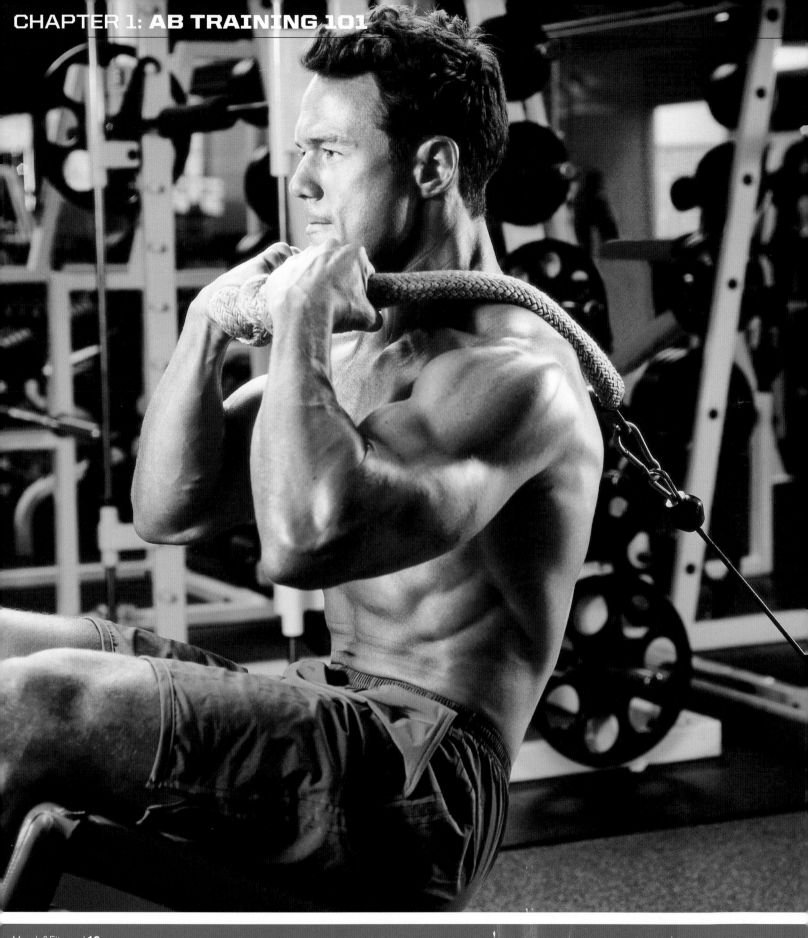

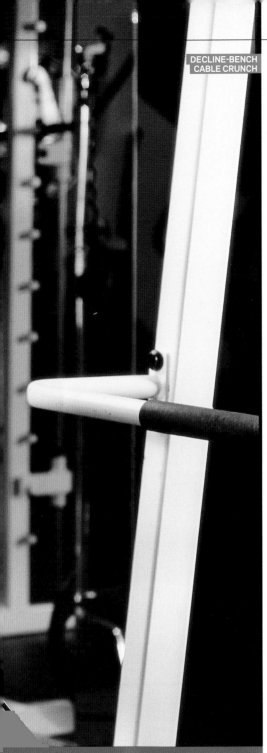

DECLINE-BENCH CABLE CRUNCH

# ROUTE 6 (PACK)

The four muscles that make up the abdominals are the rectus abdominis, the internal and external obliques, and the transverse abdominis. Without question, the best ab program is one that incorporates exercises that focus on all of these areas.

If you train abs more often than other body parts, you're not alone. Most people who give their abs the attention they deserve train them 3-5 times per week while working other major body parts (chest, back, legs, etc.) 1-3 times per week. Reason being, the abs are postural muscles that stay flexed for long periods to support the spine. As such, they have a higher percentage of slow-twitch muscle fibers than other body parts and require more regular training for adequate stimulation.

The rep range you choose to work within is critical to how your abs develop (and show) when your body fat is low. Using your own body weight as resistance and keeping your reps between 15 and 30, for example, will help you maintain a flat and lean midsection, allowing your waist to appear smaller. If you feel your abs need to grow so you can see them better, you'll need to include weighted exercises using a cable station or a lightweight plate or dumbbell to help build them up. Selecting exercises is easy—choose a total of four moves each time you train abs, one for each of the different areas.

With ab training, timing is crucial: Always hit abs last in your workout. You don't want them to be fatigued before training other body parts such as back or legs because you want your abs and core to be strong and fresh to help sustain the intra-abdominal pressure necessary to protect your spine.

So let's look at each region of the abs, dissecting the anatomy, location, and function, as well as review some of our favorite exercises to get the kind of washboard midsection you've always wanted.

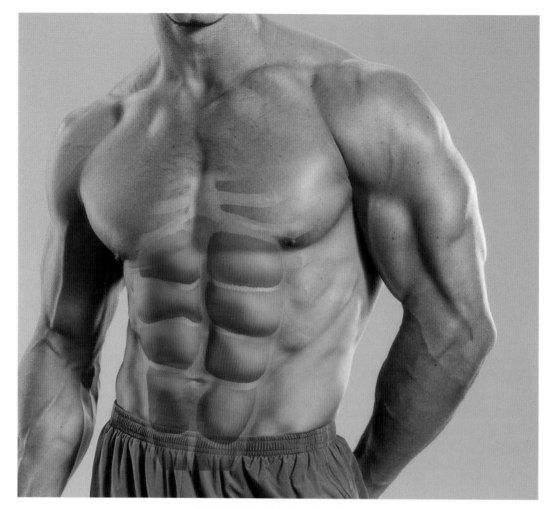

# REGION 1:
# RECTUS ABDOMINIS

Even though the six-pack looks like several individual muscles, the rectus abdominis is really only one. Running vertically from your sternum to your pelvis, the rectus is a thin sheath of muscle. While we'll discuss exercises for your upper and lower abs, note that they're all part of one muscle. That said, you can still emphasize the upper and lower portions of the rectus with specific movements.

The rectus abdominis is responsible for the standard crunching motion—moving your ribcage toward your pelvis. It also gets trained in the opposite direction, bringing your pelvis to your ribcage, which we refer to as a reverse crunching motion.

**>>Basic Exercises:** (Upper abs) crunch; (Lower abs) reverse crunch, hanging knee/leg raise
**>>Advanced Exercises:** (Upper abs) weighted crunch, machine crunch, decline bench cable crunch, kneeling cable crunch; (Lower abs) exercise-ball pull-in, dumbbell hip thrust, weighted hanging leg raise; (Upper and lower) double crunch

**DECLINE BENCH CABLE CRUNCH**
Set an adjustable bench to a moderate decline and place it in front of a low-pulley cable with a rope attachment. Sit squarely on it, feet secured under the ankle pads. Lie back on the bench and grasp the ends of the rope with your hands at the sides of your head. Contract your abs to curl your body up to a point just short of perpendicular to the floor; try to avoid pulling through your hip flexors. Round your back as you rise to increase the abdominal contraction, then lower yourself under control back to the start position.

**DUMBBELL HIP THRUST**
Lie faceup on the floor with your hands extended at your sides. Lift your feet so your legs are roughly perpendicular to the floor and place a dumbbell between your feet. (Due to the weight's placement above your body, use extra caution during this move to avoid injury.) Contract your abs to raise your hips and glutes straight up off the floor to push your feet toward the ceiling. Hold this position for a count before lowering your glutes back to the floor.

**WEIGHTED HANGING KNEE RAISE**
Perform this exercise either hanging from a high bar (using straps is an option) or on a vertical bench that supports your forearms. Hang at arm's length using an overhand grip, bending your knees 90 degrees and locking them in this position for the entire set. Hold a medicine ball between your knees or ankles. Without swinging your body, contract your abs to bring your knees toward your chest (at least above parallel to the floor) and lower under control, coming to a complete stop at the bottom so as not to generate momentum as you go into the next rep.

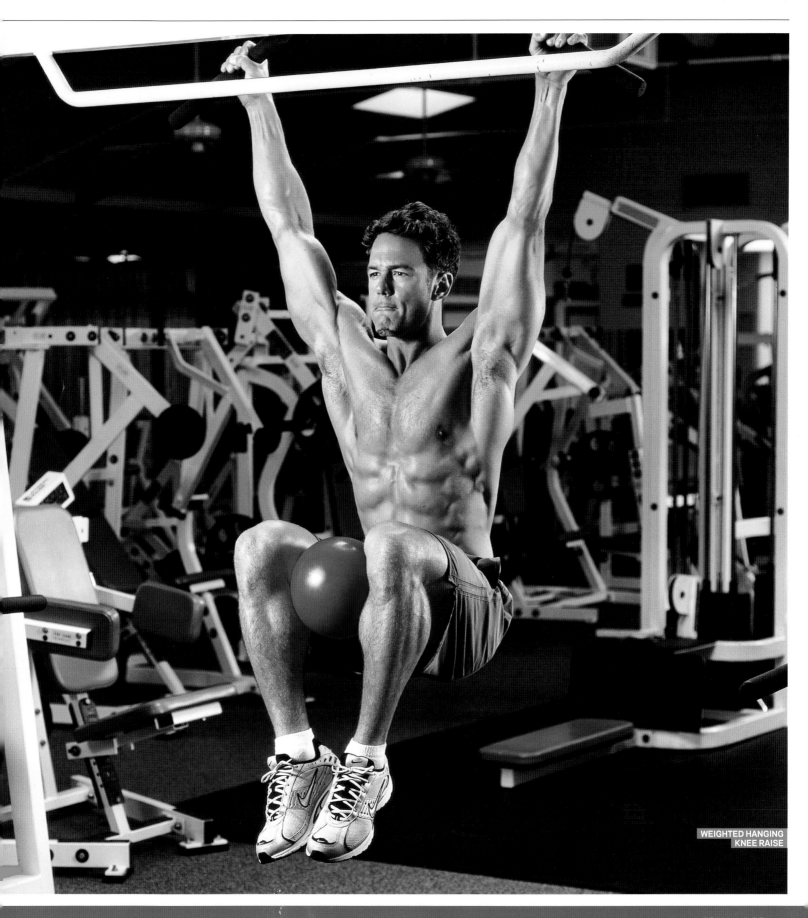

WEIGHTED HANGING
KNEE RAISE

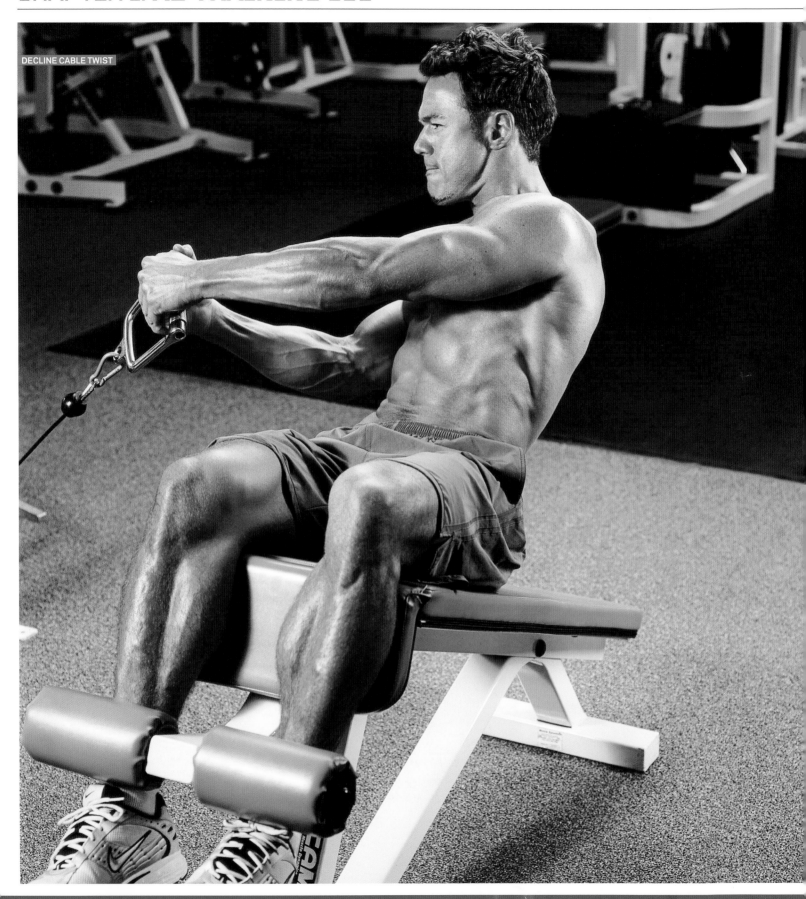

DECLINE CABLE TWIST

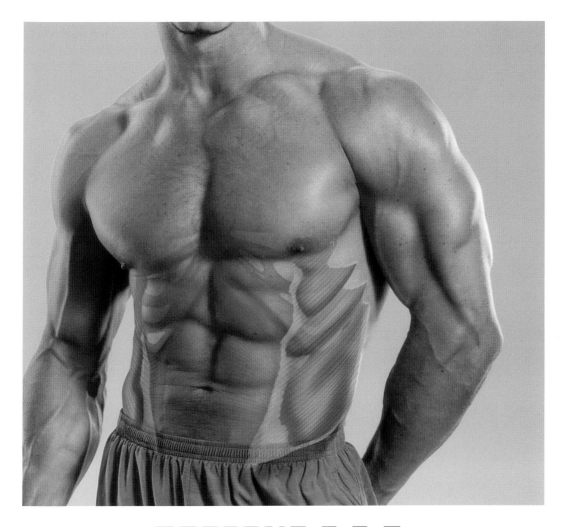

# REGIONS 2 & 3:
# INTERNAL & EXTERNAL OBLIQUES

The obliques are off to either side of the rectus abdominis and run diagonally from your lower ribs to near your hipbone. The external obliques are the ones you can see, as they're superficial to the internal obliques, which are hidden underneath. The internal and external fibers run in opposite directions. Both the internal and external obliques are responsible for torso rotation and lateral flexion of the torso.

>>**Basic Exercises:** Lying crossover crunch, oblique crunch, jackknife
>>**Advanced Exercises:** Oblique crunch on back-extension bench, standing oblique cable crunch, decline cable Russian twist

**DECLINE CABLE TWIST**
Place a decline bench in front of a cable stack with a D-handle attached to the low-pulley cable.
Sit on the bench in a half situp position (your lower back shouldn't touch down) and hold the D-handle with both hands straight above you. With your arms locked in that position, rotate your torso to the right until your right arm is about parallel to the floor. Pause for a moment, return to the start, then repeat to the left side. That's one rep.

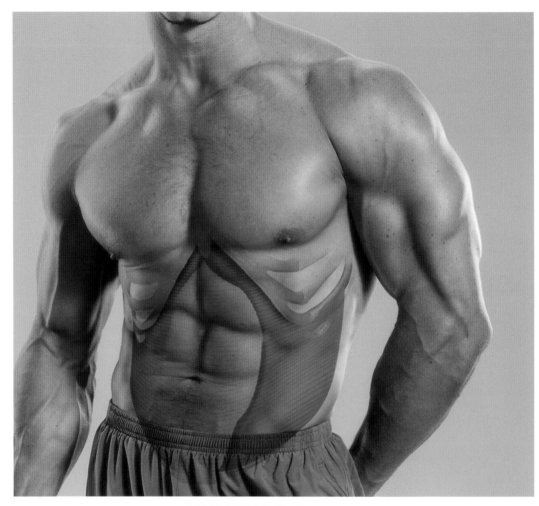

# REGION 4:
# TRANSVERSE ABDOMINIS

The transverse abdominis lies beneath the rectus abdominis, and whereas the rectus fibers run vertically, the transverse fibers run horizontally. The main function of the transverse abdominis is initiating abdominal compression during an intense exhale. You'll find this function very useful during core exercises such as the plank, where you need to keep your navel drawn in tight, as well as in moves such as the woodchop and Russian twist.

>>**Basic Exercises:** Woodchop, lying leg raise
>>**Advanced Exercises:** Exercise ball roll-out, weighted plank

**WEIGHTED PLANK**
Lie facedown on the floor with your body straight and arms extended in front of you. Have someone place a 25- to 45-pound plate on your lower back. Slowly lift your body off the floor onto your elbows and toes. Keep your abs pulled in tight and your back flat while holding this position for 30 seconds to begin with, then work toward longer periods.

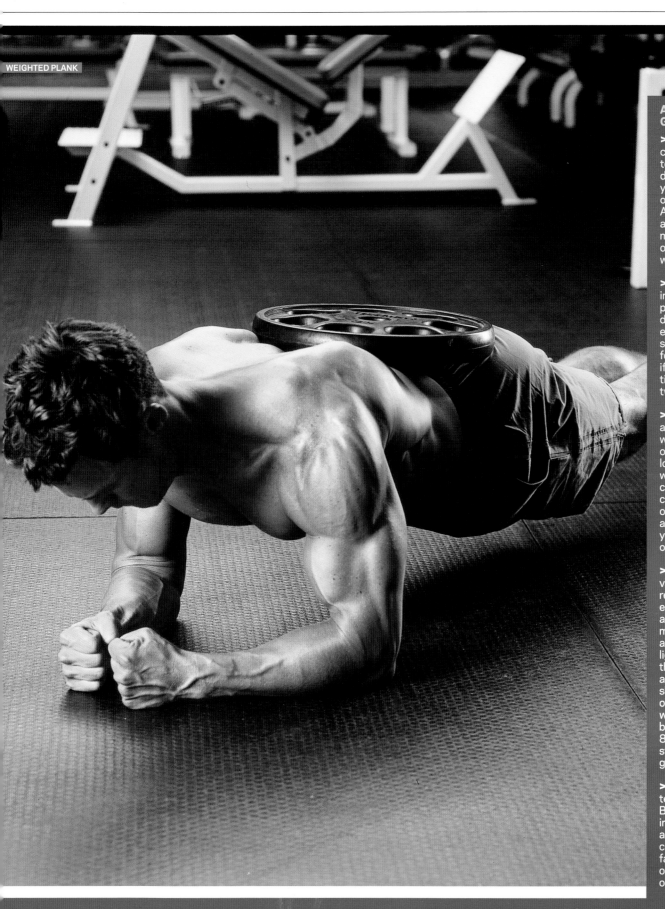

WEIGHTED PLANK

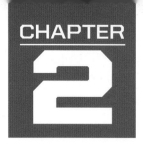

# CHAPTER 2

# 5 WEEKS TO WASHBOARD ABS

**A harder, more shredded midsection can be yours in just over a month with this training plan.**

**H**umans are creatures of habit, doing certain things over and over again because they feel comfortable, such as eating regularly at a favorite restaurant, driving the same route to work, or doing the same exercise, set, and rep schemes for a particular body part. Unfortunately, that last habit is a big problem. Getting into a rut with any muscle group isn't good, but it may be especially troublesome for abs. You don't need a Ph.D. in exercise physiology to know that making a muscle grow bigger and stronger requires continually taxing it with heavier loads or more repetitions; yet many of us often squeak by on a few sets of crunches tacked on to the end of a workout. Three sets, 20 reps each, rest, and repeat.

This five-week program solves both problems, breaking you out of a rut and introducing progression to your middle-management plan in the form of the weights you use, reps you complete, and your rest periods between sets. Building well-defined abdominals doesn't happen by accident; it takes hard work and a carefully planned approach. Operating in a comfort zone may suffice in your personal and professional lives, but if you're after a ripped sixer, complacency is your enemy. Break the pattern right now.

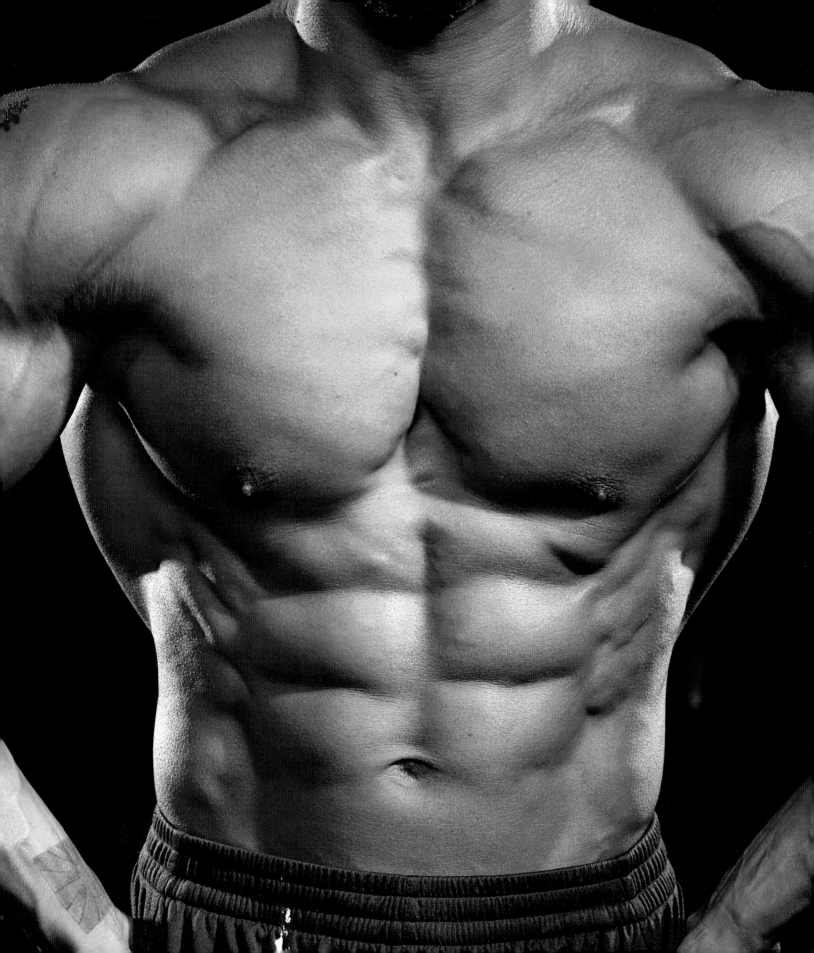

# Slam-Dunk Guidelines

Our five-week plan requires you to train your midsection three times a week, resting at least 48 hours between sessions. If possible, do abs on days you're not training a major body part.

>> **Choose one Group A exercise.** This group includes one move for each of the major regions of the abdominals—upper abs, lower abs, and obliques. Group A exercises add resistance to your body weight, meaning they're the most challenging moves in the workout and should be done early when you're fresh. Since resistance levels can be manipulated one plate at a time, even beginner-level bodybuilders can perform these moves using a lighter weight.

The key to this exercise is to choose a weight with which you can do only 10 reps, to focus on building strength in your abs. If you can't complete 10, the weight's too heavy; conversely, if you can do more than 10, the weight's too light. Selecting the right resistance is critical to manipulating intensity during the program.

>> **Choose one Group B exercise.** These intermediate-level exercises are slightly easier than Group A moves. Some Group B movements use added resistance—again, manipulate loads to fit your needs if you're a beginner.

Like Group A, this group has one exercise dedicated to lower abs, one for upper abs, and one for obliques. Although you may want to alternate which area of the abs you focus on as you progress through a workout, it's not required. In fact, one way to prevent the abdominals from becoming accustomed to a particular mode of training is to keep changing up the order of the moves.

The key with the second exercise is to choose a level of difficulty (via resistance or body position) that enables you to complete exactly 15 reps. The higher rep target works the abs in a slightly different way than that of the Group A move, building the ridges and valleys that make up a taut midsection. Hence, choosing the right resistance is an important factor in allowing you to achieve the target rep goal.

>> **Choose a Group C exercise.** These are beginner-oriented body-weight-only moves, but if you've been training hard thus far, they'll still be challenging. Again, there's one exercise for upper abs, one for lower abs, and one for obliques, so the one you choose should be determined by which areas you've trained so far and what you want to focus on.

These moves turn up the fire even more by working in a higher rep zone. Aim for 20 reps per set; if that's too easy, we list ways to make them more difficult under each exercise description. At the higher rep range, your abs will feel the burn much sooner, as you train them in a slightly different manner to emphasize muscle endurance.

>> **Rest periods for ab training vary by individual, but start with a timed 60-second interval to determine if that's adequate.** The abdominals are a fairly small muscle group that recovers quickly and doesn't require the same amount of rest between sets as larger body parts do. You don't want them to recover fully before the next set.

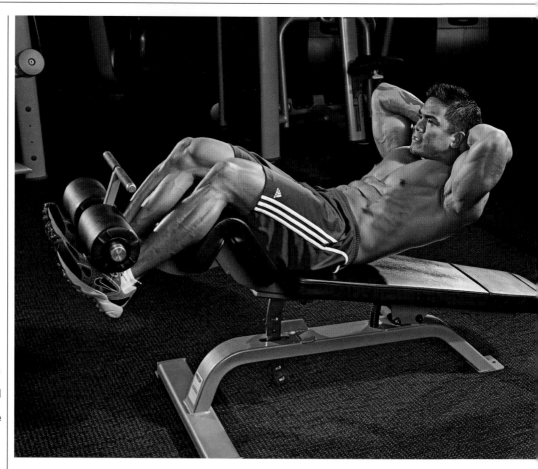

>> At your next ab-training session that week, select an exercise from each group you did not perform in the previous training session(s). If you did the lower ab machine from Group A on Tuesday, pick one of the other two Group A moves on Thursday. On your last abdominal training day that week, perform the remaining exercise. This strategy ensures that all areas of your abs get worked first when your energy levels are highest and through all the training zones: heavy for 10 reps to focus on strength, moderate for 15 reps to build size, and with body-weight only for 20 reps to make the abs burn and build muscle endurance.

# The Next Level

We promised an ab workout that accounts for progression over time—that is, as your abs become stronger, you want to keep challenging them for continued progress. Here's how you'll do that in Week 2 and beyond:

>> On all Group A moves, add one plate each week and still try to complete 10 reps per set. Increasing the resistance weekly makes the abs work harder. If you can't do 10 reps, no problem—the key is to increase the weight and try to do as many reps as you can. This is why choosing the right weight in Week 1 is so important. Do this on all three sets for all Group A exercises.

>> On Group B moves, reduce the rest period between sets by five seconds each week. During Week 2, rest just 55 seconds between sets. The third week,

reduce the rest interval by another five seconds. Continue in this manner until you're resting only 40 seconds by the fifth week. Progressively limiting your rest period is another way to increase the intensity of your workout and make your abs stronger and more efficient. You're still trying to reach the 15-rep target on every set for Group B exercises.

>> On Group C moves, perform one additional rep each week, keeping the resistance and rest intervals the same as in Week 1. In the second week, do 21 reps instead of 20, and increase that by one rep each week. By the fifth week, you're doing 24 reps for all sets of each Group C exercise.

# Dial It In

While the keys that drive our five-week program are variety and progression, it would be a mistake to think that's all that's required to build washboard abs. Pay particular attention to your diet—monitoring carb and fat intake and total calories, and following a smart supplementation program—while including four 30-minute cardio sessions a week to strip off body fat. Only through a combination of these elements can you truly bring out a ripped six-pack.

At the end of five weeks, your abs will be much improved—and the proof will be in the mirror as well as in your advancing strength. You can return to this program at a future date, but it's not intended to be followed indefinitely. Just make sure whatever plan you follow challenges you.

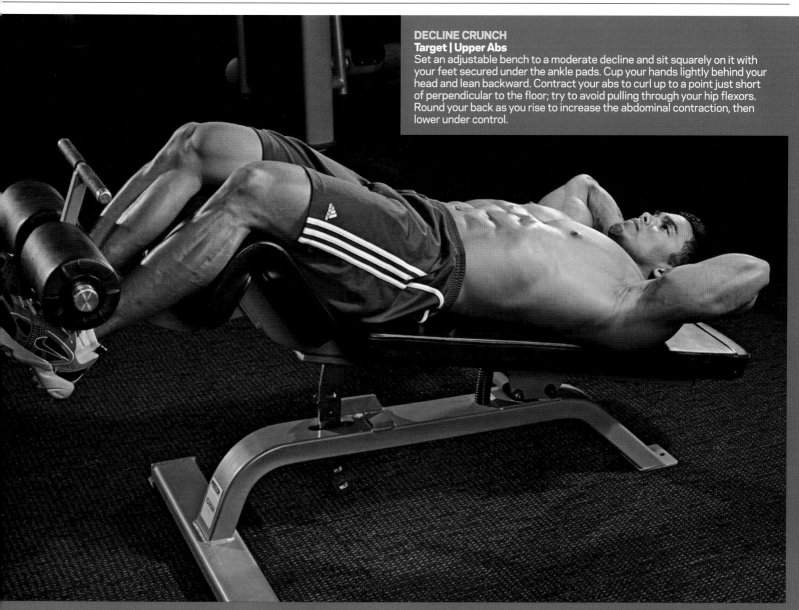

## DECLINE CRUNCH
**Target | Upper Abs**

Set an adjustable bench to a moderate decline and sit squarely on it with your feet secured under the ankle pads. Cup your hands lightly behind your head and lean backward. Contract your abs to curl up to a point just short of perpendicular to the floor; try to avoid pulling through your hip flexors. Round your back as you rise to increase the abdominal contraction, then lower under control.

# PERFORMANCE POINTERS

**1)** Hold the peak contraction. By consciously squeezing and momentarily holding at the top of each rep, you'll work your abdominals harder and be less inclined to race through your repetitions.

**2)** Move at a smooth, deliberate pace. Use a slow, strict motion that increases the intensity of the contraction and minimizes momentum. Momentum is created using fast, explosive motions, which reduce the quality of your workout and invite injury.

**3)** Exhale at the top of the move. Hold your breath until you have reached the peak-contracted position for a stronger, more intense contraction. Exhaling early reduces intra-abdominal pressure, so you won't be able to contract your abs as strongly.

**4)** Keep your head in line with your torso. When grasping your head to support it, don't interlock your fingers, which increases the likelihood you'll pull on your head and disrupt spinal alignment. Instead, lightly cup your fingers behind your head to support it.

**5)** Make sure the action is restricted to your waist. During most upper- and lower-abdominal moves, your spine flexes (your lower back rounds), so keep your lower back as flat as possible, not arched, during the movements. Keep other joints stabilized.

**6)** The range of motion is fairly small in many abdominal moves. Bringing your shoulder blades off the floor in the basic crunch, for example, works the abs through a full range of motion. Don't rise as high as you would in a full situp—such motion doesn't further contract or stimulate the abs but may increase hip flexor involvement when your feet are planted, such as in decline-bench crunches.

**7)** Maintain constant tension throughout the set. The ab muscles recover quickly, so if you rest between reps, even if for only a second, it becomes difficult to adequately fatigue the muscle. Maintain constant tension by stopping just short of the endpoint on the eccentric rep.

**8)** Take precise rest periods between sets. After you complete your set, rest about 60 seconds to let your abs recover so you can complete your next set. If you start too early, they'll still be fatigued and you won't reach your target rep.

# GROUP A: STRENGTH BUILDERS

>> Choose one of these three Group A exercises, which are considered advanced moves because you can add resistance simply by changing the pin on the weight stack. Be sure to fine-tune the resistance so you hit the target rep (10) by adding/subtracting weight. For your ab workouts later that same week, choose one of the other moves each time. (Note: If you're less advanced, simply use a lighter resistance with which you can complete the recommended number of sets and reps.)

**SETS + REPS | Do three** sets of 10 reps the first week. Over the course of the next five weeks, add one plate (about 10 pounds) each week (so that by Week 5 you've added four plates), still trying to reach 10 reps but doing as many as you can.

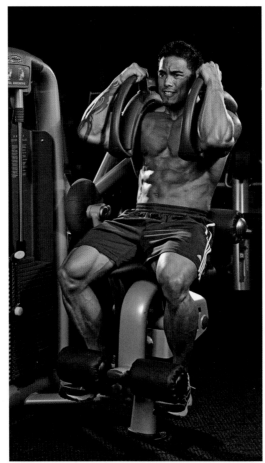

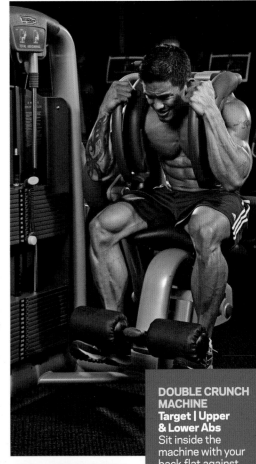

### DOUBLE CRUNCH MACHINE
**Target | Upper & Lower Abs**
Sit inside the machine with your back flat against the pad. Hook your feet under the ankle pads and secure the shoulder pads firmly over your upper torso. Grasp the handles with both hands. With your head in a neutral position and eyes focused forward, crunch your upper body forward while simultaneously lifting your legs toward your upper body. Hold the peak contraction, then return to the start. Don't allow the weights to touch down between reps, to keep constant tension on your abs.

### LYING CABLE CRUNCH
**Target | Upper Abs**
Lie faceup directly in front of a low-pulley cable with a rope attached, with your knees bent and feet flat on the floor. Grasp the rope with a neutral grip, placing your hands by your ears and locking your arms in this position for the duration of the set. Contract your abs to curl up as high as you can, squeezing at the top, then lower to just short of your shoulder blades resting on the floor between reps.

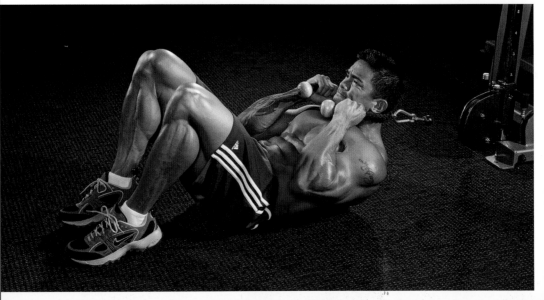

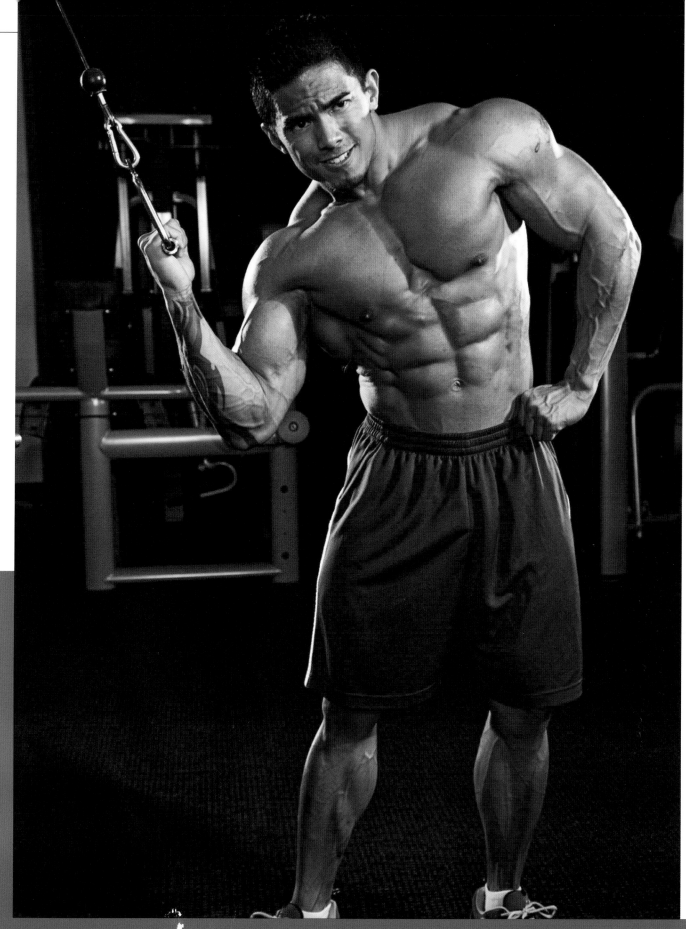

## STANDING OBLIQUE CABLE CRUNCH

**Target | Obliques**
Stand about two feet away from a cable stack, your right shoulder facing the pulley. Attach a D-handle to the high cable and grasp it with an underhand grip, bending your arm about 90 degrees and locking it in this position for the duration of the set. Using your obliques, crunch down laterally as far as you can, holding the peak contraction briefly. Complete all reps for one side, then switch sides.

# GROUP B:
# SIZE BUILDERS

>> Choose one of these three Group B exercises, which are considered intermediate moves. Again, fine-tune the move to hit the target reps (15): For the decline-bench crunch, increase or decrease the angle of the bench; for the hanging knee raise, increase or decrease the bend in your knees; for the cable woodchop, add/subtract resistance. Select a different move for the week's second session, then do the remaining exercise in the final workout.

**SETS + REPS |** Perform three sets of 15 reps the first week. Over the course of the next five weeks, reduce your rest period between sets by five seconds each week (so by Week 3, you've cut 10 seconds off your rest period), still trying to do 15 reps each set. After five weeks, return to the normal rest period with which you can perform 15 reps—at this point, you should be able to do a more challenging variation of the move than when you started.

### DECLINE CRUNCH
**Target | Upper Abs**
Set an adjustable bench to a moderate decline and sit squarely on it, with your feet secured under the ankle pads. Cup your hands lightly behind your head and lean backward. Contract your abs to curl up to a point just short of perpendicular to the floor; try to avoid pulling through your hip flexors. Round your back as you rise to increase the abdominal contraction, then lower under control.

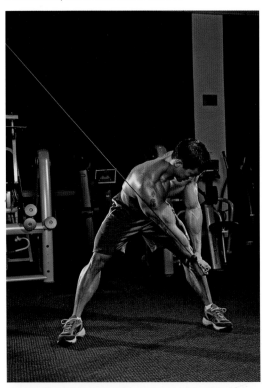

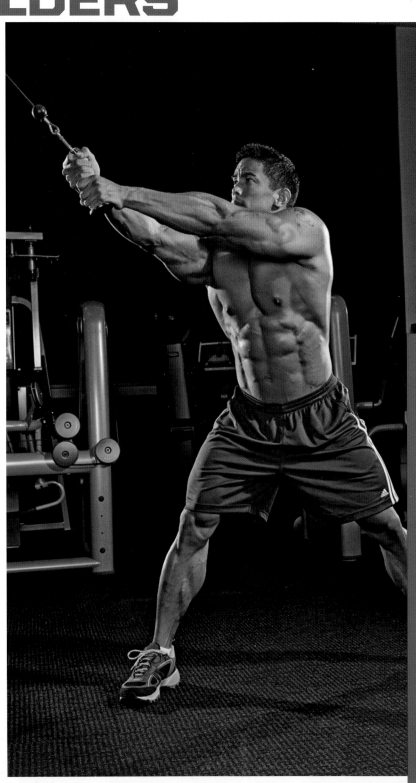

### CABLE WOODCHOP
**Target | Upper Abs, Obliques**
Stand erect with your feet outside shoulder width and knees slightly bent alongside a high-pulley cable (with a D-handle or I-handle attached), your right shoulder facing the pulley. Reach across your body with your left hand and grasp the handle, placing your right hand on top. Keep your arms straight but unlocked throughout the set. Rotate your torso at the waist to the left by contracting your left obliques, pulling the handle down in an arc across your body to a position just below your knee. Keep your left arm as straight as possible. Return and repeat for reps. Do both sides.

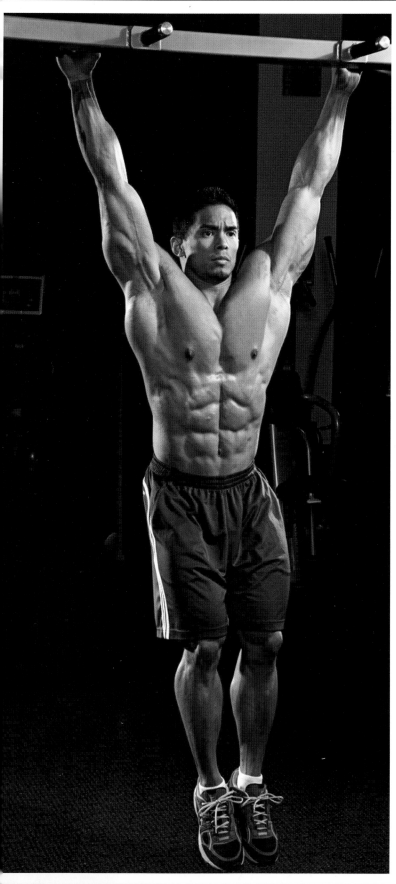
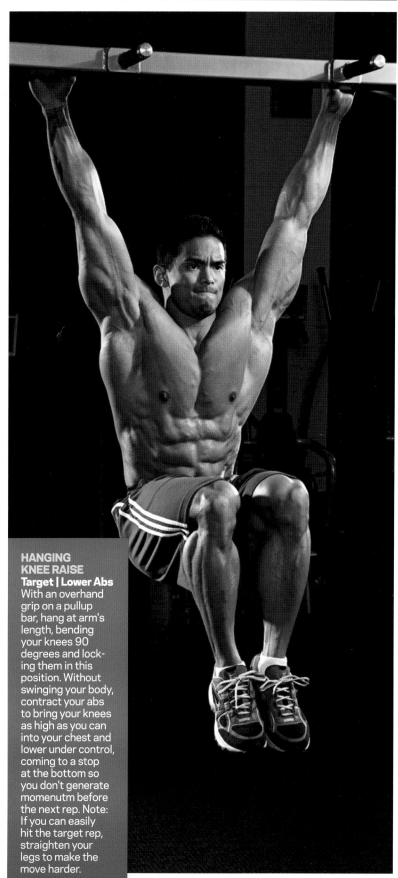

**HANGING KNEE RAISE**

**Target | Lower Abs**

With an overhand grip on a pullup bar, hang at arm's length, bending your knees 90 degrees and locking them in this position. Without swinging your body, contract your abs to bring your knees as high as you can into your chest and lower under control, coming to a stop at the bottom so you don't generate momenutm before the next rep. Note: If you can easily hit the target rep, straighten your legs to make the move harder.

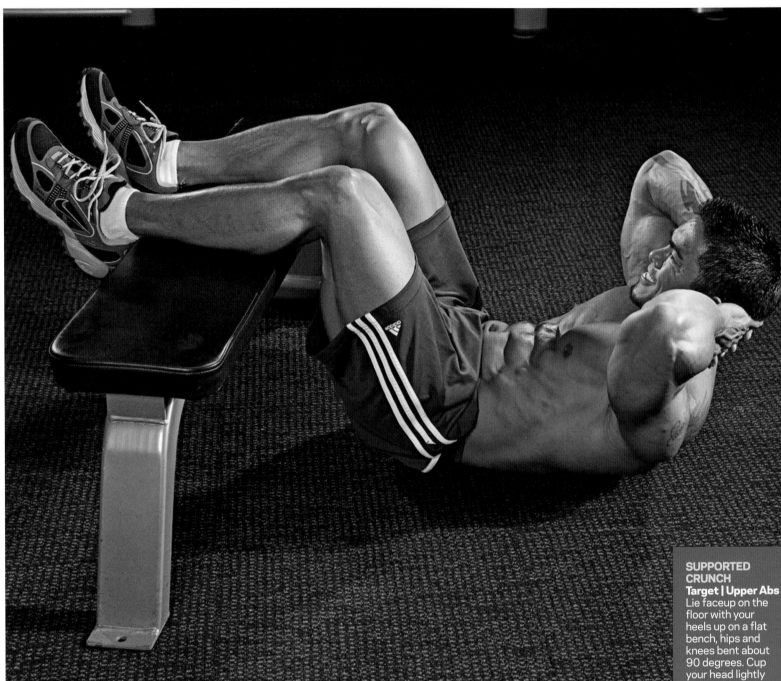

# GROUP C:
# ENDURANCE BUILDERS

>> Select one of these three Group C exercises, which are considered beginner moves, done with just your body weight. Again, make slight adjustments in how you perform each exercise to fine-tune the degree of difficulty so you hit the target rep. For your next two ab sessions that week, choose one of the other moves each time.

SETS + REPS | Do three sets of 20 reps the first week. Over the course of the next five weeks, strive to do one more repetition per set each week so that after five weeks you do 24 reps on each set (keeping the resistance and the rest periods unchanged). After five weeks, increase the level of difficulty of each move as you start again at 20 reps per set.

**SUPPORTED CRUNCH**
**Target | Upper Abs**
Lie faceup on the floor with your heels up on a flat bench, hips and knees bent about 90 degrees. Cup your head lightly with your hands. Contract your abs to rise as high as you can, bringing your shoulder blades off the floor without pulling on your head. Lower under control. Note: To increase the level of difficulty, don't allow your shoulder blades to touch down at the bottom of each rep.

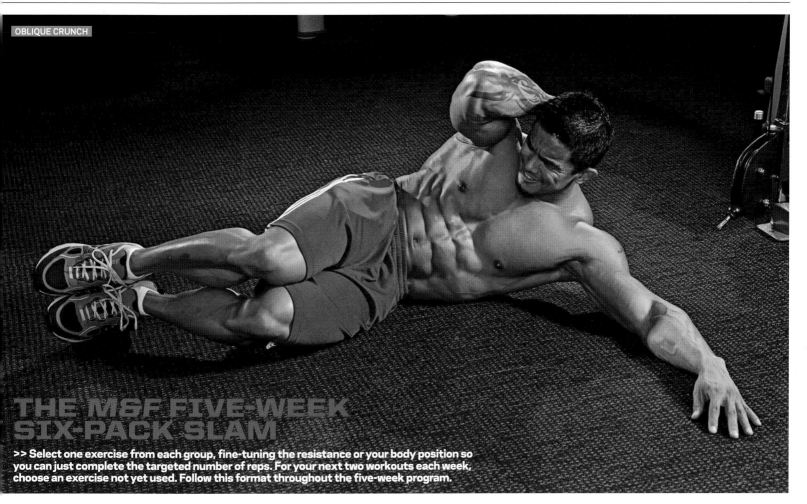

OBLIQUE CRUNCH

# THE M&F FIVE-WEEK SIX-PACK SLAM

>> Select one exercise from each group, fine-tuning the resistance or your body position so you can just complete the targeted number of reps. For your next two workouts each week, choose an exercise not yet used. Follow this format throughout the five-week program.

## GROUP A: STRENGTH BUILDERS

| Choose one: | SETS | WEEK 1 REPS | WEEK 2 REPS | WEEK 3 REPS | WEEK 4 REPS | WEEK 5 REPS |
|---|---|---|---|---|---|---|
| Double Crunch Machine | 3 | 10 | Up to 10 | Up to 10 | Up to 10 | Up to 10 |
| Lying Cable Crunch | 3 | 10 | Up to 10 | Up to 10 | Up to 10 | Up to 10 |
| Standing Oblique Cable Crunch* | 3 | 10 | Up to 10 | Up to 10 | Up to 10 | Up to 10 |

### Instructions
*Week 1: Choose a resistance with which you can complete just 10 reps.*
*Week 2: Add one plate to the weight used the previous week, trying to get the same number of reps (do as many as possible).*
*Weeks 3–5: Add one more plate to what you used in Week 2, then add another plate in Week 4, then another in Week 5.*

## GROUP B: SIZE BUILDERS

| Choose one: | SETS | WEEK 1 REPS | WEEK 2 REPS | WEEK 3 REPS | WEEK 4 REPS | WEEK 5 REPS |
|---|---|---|---|---|---|---|
| Hanging Knee Raise | 3 | 15 | Up to 15 | Up to 15 | Up to 15 | Up to 15 |
| Decline Crunch | 3 | 15 | Up to 15 | Up to 15 | Up to 15 | Up to 15 |
| Cable Woodchop* | 3 | 15 | Up to 15 | Up to 15 | Up to 15 | Up to 15 |

### Instructions
*Week 1: Choose a resistance or level of difficulty with which you can complete just 15 reps.*
*Week 2: Reduce your rest period between sets by five seconds, aiming to do the same number of reps as the week before for all sets.*
*Weeks 3–5: Reduce your between-sets rest period by another five seconds each week.*

## GROUP C: ENDURANCE BUILDERS

| Choose one: | SETS | WEEK 1 REPS | WEEK 2 REPS | WEEK 3 REPS | WEEK 4 REPS | WEEK 5 REPS |
|---|---|---|---|---|---|---|
| Reverse Crunch | 3 | 20 | 21 | 22 | 23 | 24 |
| Supported Crunch | 3 | 20 | 21 | 22 | 23 | 24 |
| Oblique Crunch* | 3 | 20 | 21 | 22 | 23 | 24 |

### Instructions
*Week 1: Choose a variation of this body-weight move that allows you to perform just 20 reps.*
*Week 2: Do one additional rep on all sets using normal rest periods and the same resistance you used in Week 1.*
*Weeks 3–5: Each week add another rep to all sets.*
*DO THE NUMBER OF REPS LISTED TO EACH SIDE.*

# CHAPTER 3

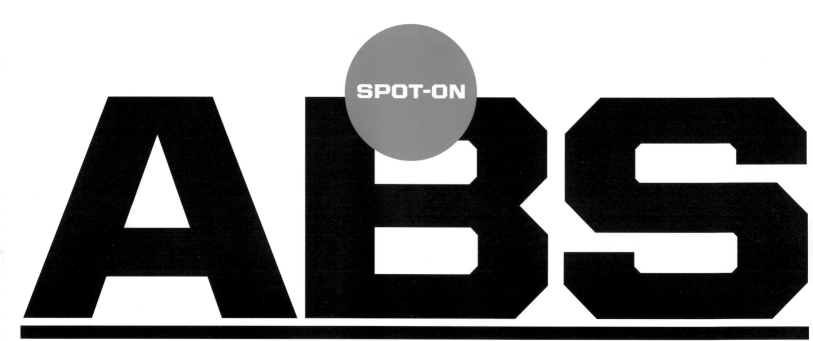

**SPOT-ON**

# ABS

## This science-based training routine will help you spot-reduce for a more chiseled midsection in six weeks.

**W**ho would you believe? The Barbie and Ken look-alikes on the infomercials who say that if you use their ab-training gizmos "You'll lose inches off your waist in just a few weeks!" or the many scientists who say such a claim is totally bogus?

After all, attaining a washboard midsection simply by doing an ab exercise for five minutes a day is more or less the definition of spot-reducing, an outdated method of fat loss that has been relegated to a weight-room punch line.

Well, now you can stop laughing—it seems the spot-reduction theory may actually hold water. Doing ab exercises for prolonged periods can, in fact, help you get better abs, and we've designed a program for you to achieve just that. All of which makes Barbie and Ken's logic, according to scientific research, brilliant!

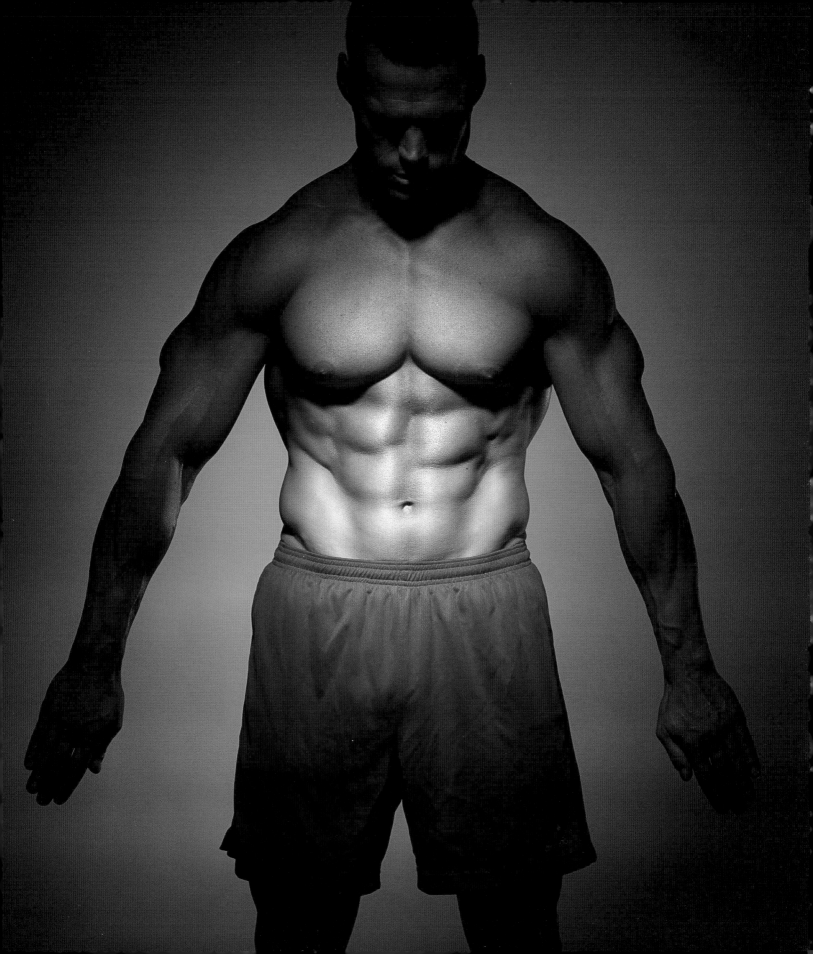

# SPOT-REDUCTION RESEARCH

OK, maybe Barbie and Ken aren't 100% correct. Although you may not be able to spot-reduce your midsection fat to reveal ripped abs by using some gizmo for just five minutes a day, you can spot-reduce your waistline with the right program.

Spot reduction refers to the ability to train a muscle group, such as abs, with region-specific exercises, such as crunches, in an effort to remove body fat from just that area of the body. Until last year, if you asked any exercise physiologist if it were possible to spot-reduce your middle, you'd get an emphatic "Hell, no!" Now, that same expert, assuming he or she has been paying attention to the latest research on the subject, would want to retract that statement.

A major study published in the *American Journal of Physiology* uncovered some interesting results, effectively turning the world of exercise science on its ear. In the study, conducted at the University of Copenhagen (Denmark), scientists had male subjects perform single-leg extensions with light weight for 30 minutes straight. The researchers then measured the amount of blood flow to the subjects' subcutaneous fat cells (those under the skin) in both the exercising and resting thighs, as well as the amount of lipolysis (release of fat) from those fat cells. The scientists discovered that the exercising leg experienced a significant increase in blood flow to and lipolysis from the subcutaneous fat cells, compared with the resting leg. In other words, during exercise, the fat cells surrounding the trained muscle released more fat into the blood, meaning a greater quantity of fat is fed to the exercising muscles to be used as fuel.

The results of the study suggest that when you exercise, you do, in fact, burn body fat preferentially from the area you're training. Although the study looked at fat on the thighs, it's safe to assume that these results will hold up when you perform exercises for your abs and oblique muscles.

In addition, the findings of numerous studies indicate that exercise programs, particularly those that combine weights and cardio, are very effective at reducing fat from all areas of the body, especially the abdominal and visceral fat that lies beneath the ab muscles and is responsible for the "beer belly" many middle-aged men develop. Outside of being unattractive, this fat is directly related to heart disease, research shows.

The good news for those of you already lifting and doing cardio is that you're ahead of the game. Combine those elements with a program specifically designed to melt the fat off your midsection, like the one in this article, and by the time summer rolls around you'll have changed that potential pony keg into a six-pack.

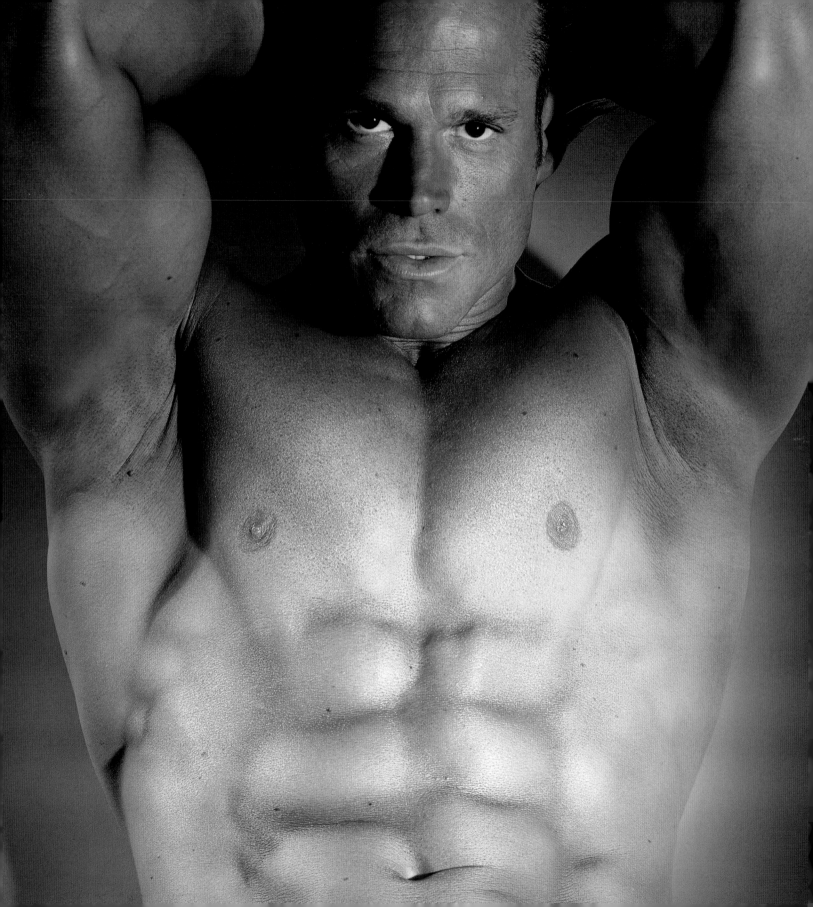

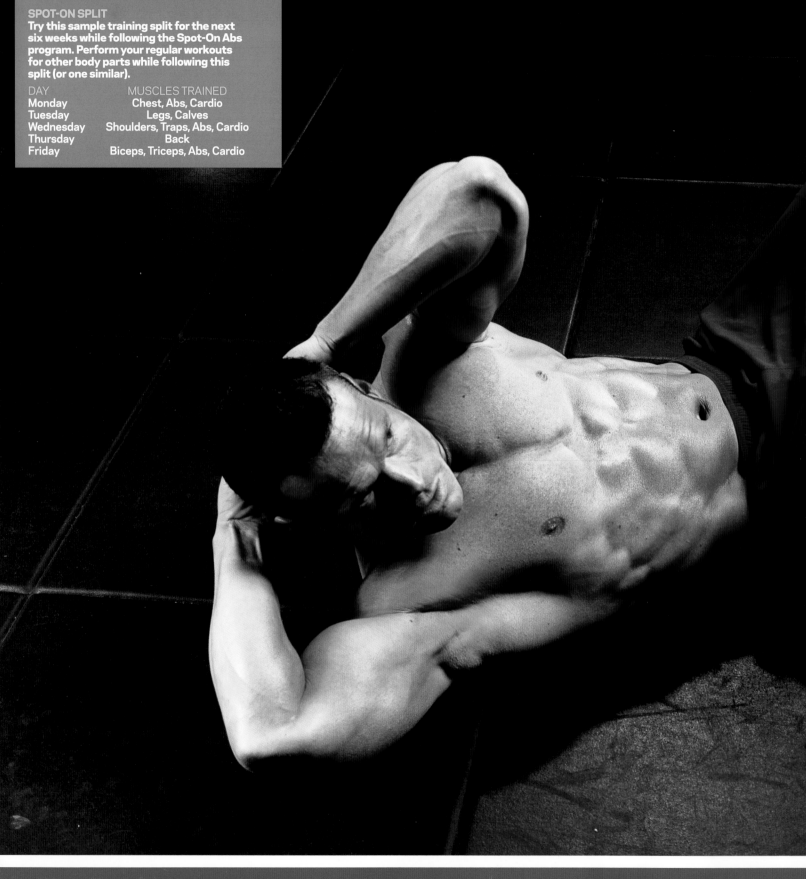

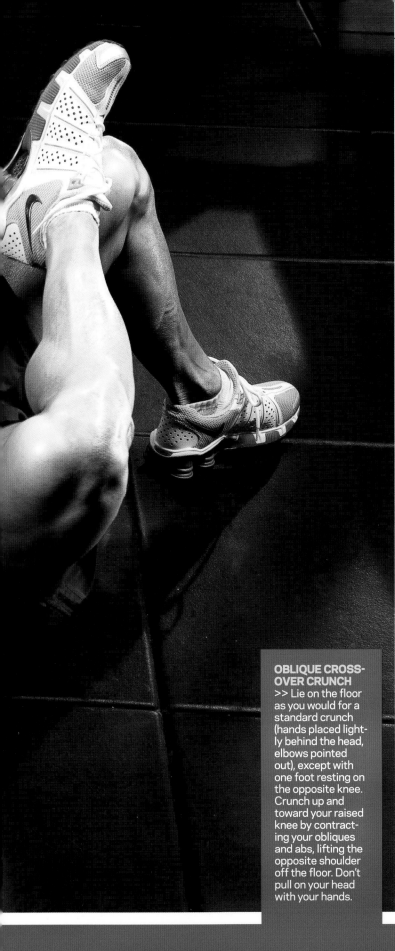

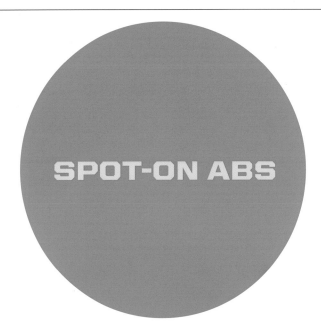

# SPOT-ON ABS

The Spot-On Abs program is different from your typical ab routine because each workout is based on total time, not reps and sets. The Danish study had subjects train with light weight for 30 minutes. Therefore, similar to the study protocol, you'll work your abs in giant-set fashion, moving from one exercise to the next (four to seven exercises total per workout) with little, if any, rest for a specific period.

During the first week of this six- week program, you'll perform four ab exercises continuously for 15 minutes straight, meaning you'll do one set after another with little to no rest in between. Perform each set with strict form and at a medium pace; don't try to do the reps too fast, because it's length of time you're going for, not a particular number of sets or reps. (How many sets actually completed in the allotted time will vary by individual.) In Week 2, you'll do five exercises for 20 minutes; in Weeks 3 and 4, six exercises for 25 minutes; and in Weeks 5 and 6, seven exercises for 30 minutes. Following each ab workout, you'll perform 30 minutes of cardio on a treadmill.

During Week 1, shoot for 10 reps per set and no more. This will be very easy for the majority of the exercises at the start of the workout, but keep in mind, you're cycling these exercises with little to no rest between sets. After the first five minutes, 10 reps will become difficult, if not impossible, to complete. (If you can't make it to 10, just do as many reps as possible.) During Week 2, bump up the reps to 12 per set, as your abdominal conditioning should be improving. Of course, you have an extra five minutes of ab work to do this week. During Weeks 3 and 4, aim for 15 reps per set; Weeks 5 and 6 call for 20 reps. Be sure to rest no more than 15 seconds between exercises—the goal is to keep moving to maximize fat-burning.

Perform these ab routines three times a week at the end of your regular workouts. We suggest doing them on Monday, Wednesday, and Friday to allow adequate recovery between sessions. Continue training other muscle groups as you normally do; however, since you're training abs Monday, Wednesday, and Friday, we also recommend that you follow a five-day, Monday through Friday training split and take the weekend off, as in the "Spot-On Split" sidebar.

Cardio should be done on a treadmill, if possible, as this has been shown to be just about the most effective form of cardio for maximizing the amount of fat burned. Another way to get the most out of fat-melting is to perform your cardio in the following manner: After a two-minute warmup, get into high gear and do high-intensity cardio (about 85% of your maximum heart rate, or MHR) in the first half of your workout, then reduce the intensity (about 60% MHR) during the second half. (See "Spotty Cardio" sidebar for a sample cardio workout following this method.) Not only does research show that this type of cardio activity burns more fat during a workout, but higher-intensity cardio has also been found to burn the most fat after training is over—and that, after all, is the ultimate goal.

Is this program grueling? Yes. But do you want abs by the time summer is here, or would you prefer spending another vacation wearing a tank top at the beach to flaunt your guns and hide your no-show abs? Thought so.

**OBLIQUE CROSS-OVER CRUNCH**
>> Lie on the floor as you would for a standard crunch (hands placed lightly behind the head, elbows pointed out), except with one foot resting on the opposite knee. Crunch up and toward your raised knee by contracting your obliques and abs, lifting the opposite shoulder off the floor. Don't pull on your head with your hands.

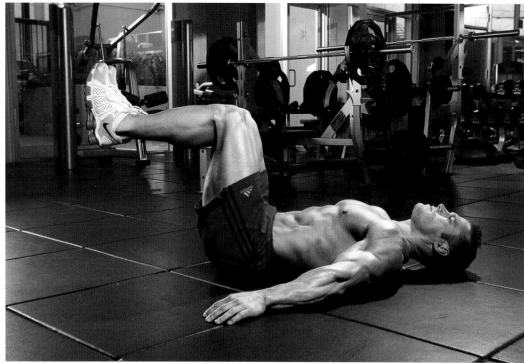

# SPOT-ON ABS PROGRAM

These workouts become more challenging as the weeks go by, progressively conditioning your abs so they can handle the highest volume of training during Weeks 5 and 6. Remember, it's not about how many total sets you complete (this will vary from person to person) but rather that you're able to perform sets one after the other for the entire period specified. For all exercises, keep your technique strict and move at a medium pace—don't hurry.

## WEEK 1

Do each of the following exercises for 10 reps (or until you reach failure) in giant-set fashion (doing the exercises one after another without resting between each) for 15 minutes:

*Reverse Crunch*
*Crunch*
*Oblique Crunch*
*Rope Crunch*

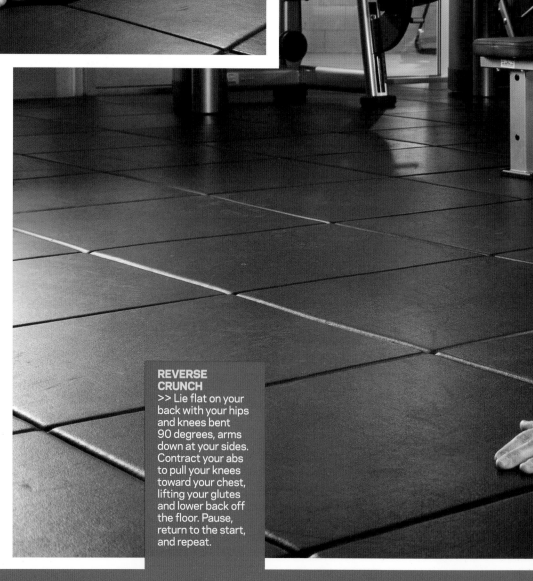

**REVERSE CRUNCH**
>> Lie flat on your back with your hips and knees bent 90 degrees, arms down at your sides. Contract your abs to pull your knees toward your chest, lifting your glutes and lower back off the floor. Pause, return to the start, and repeat.

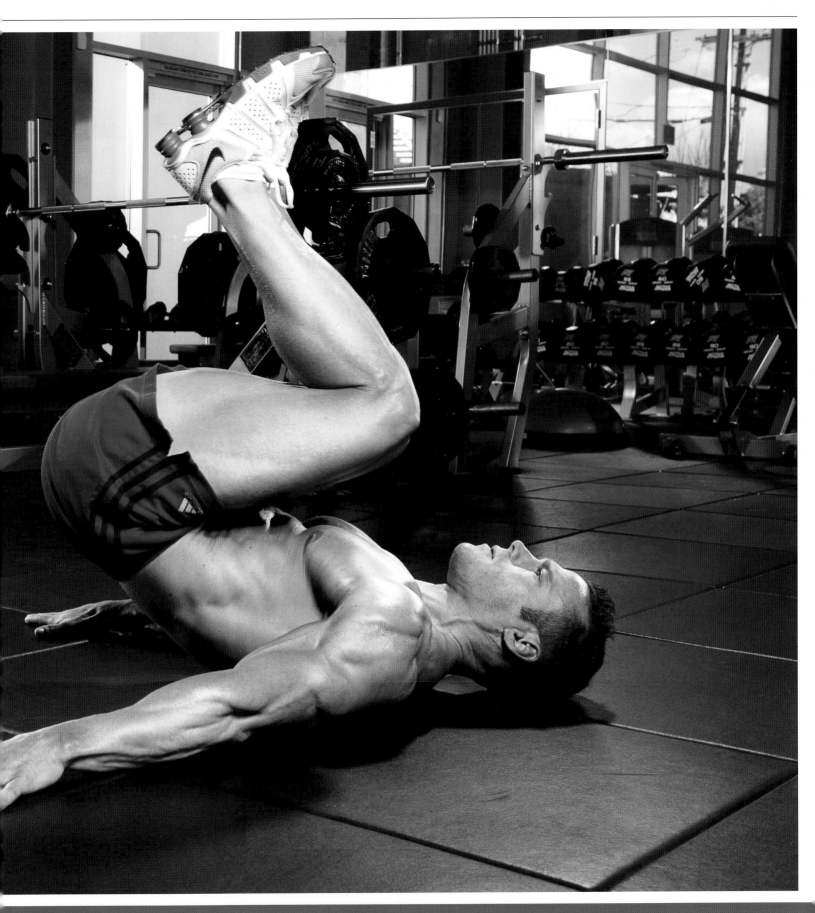

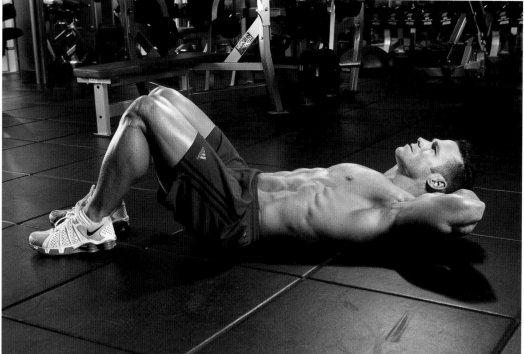

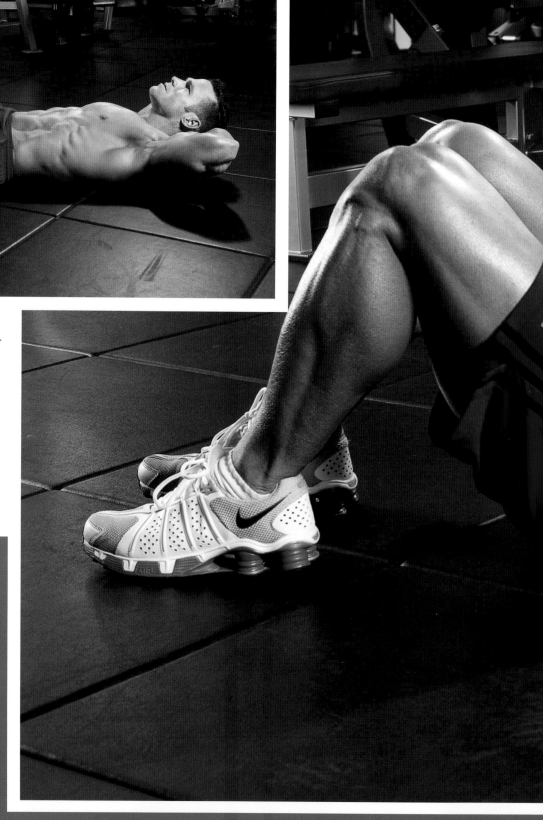

## WEEK 2
**Do each of the following exercises for 12 reps (or until failure) in giant-set fashion for 20 minutes:**

*Hanging Knee Raise*
*Reverse Crunch*
*Crunch*
*Oblique Crunch*
*Rope Crunch*

### CRUNCH
>> Lie flat on your back with your knees bent and place your hands lightly behind your head. Crunch up by contracting your abs, raising your shoulder blades off the floor. Hold the contraction for a count at the top before lowering.

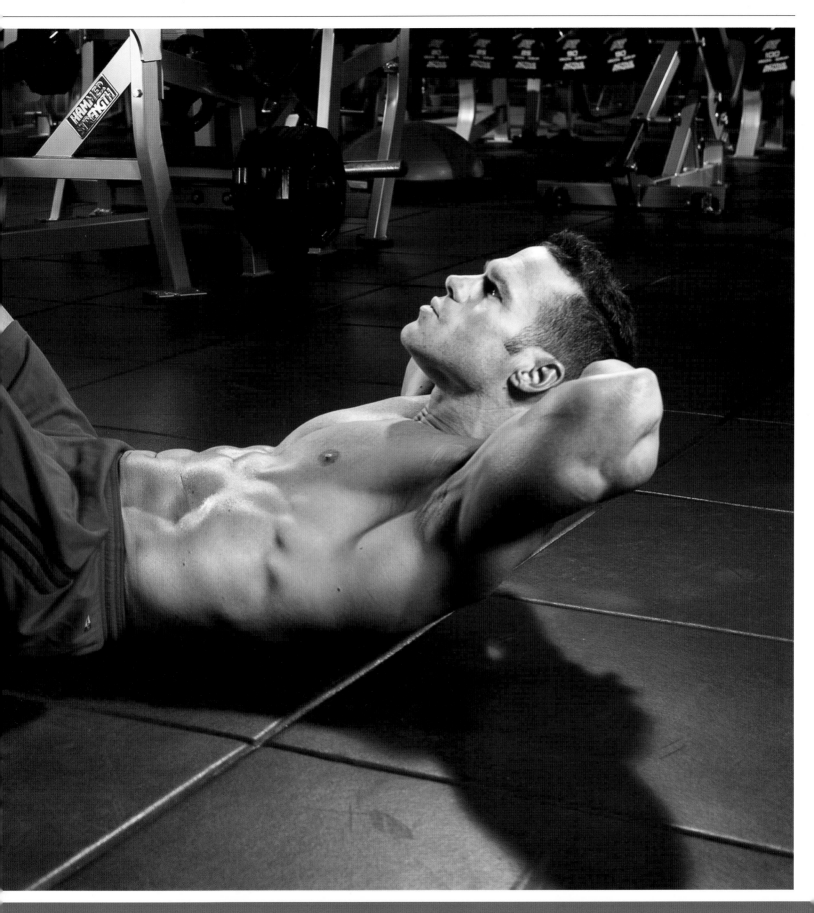

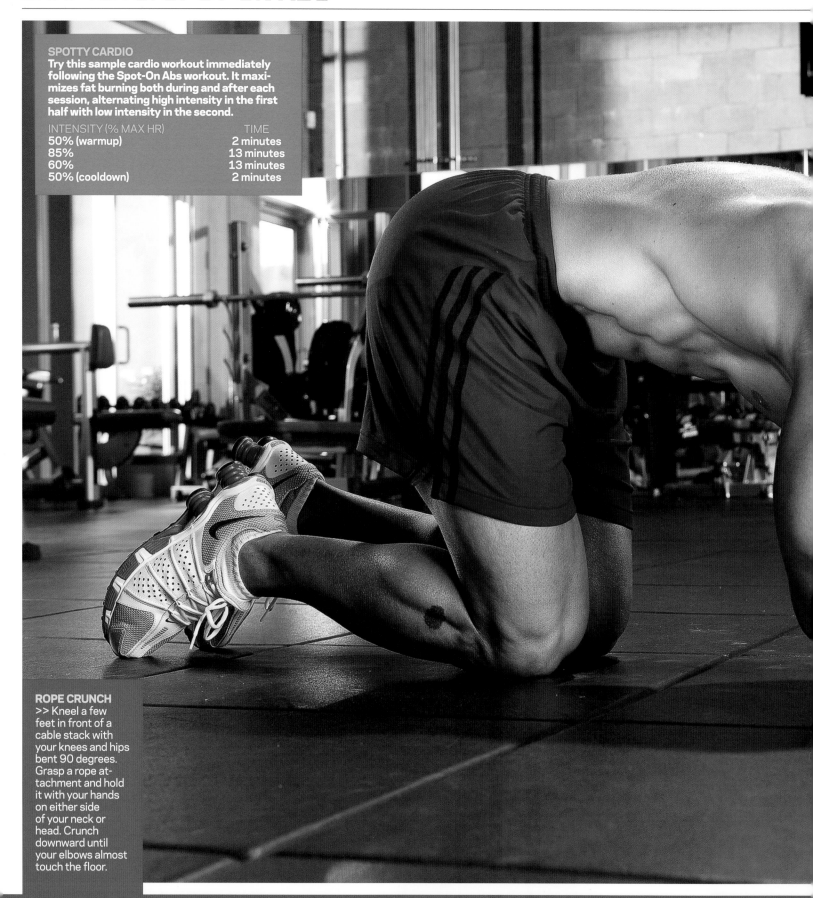

## SPOTTY CARDIO

Try this sample cardio workout immediately following the Spot-On Abs workout. It maximizes fat burning both during and after each session, alternating high intensity in the first half with low intensity in the second.

| INTENSITY (% MAX HR) | TIME |
|---|---|
| 50% (warmup) | 2 minutes |
| 85% | 13 minutes |
| 60% | 13 minutes |
| 50% (cooldown) | 2 minutes |

## ROPE CRUNCH

>> Kneel a few feet in front of a cable stack with your knees and hips bent 90 degrees. Grasp a rope attachment and hold it with your hands on either side of your neck or head. Crunch downward until your elbows almost touch the floor.

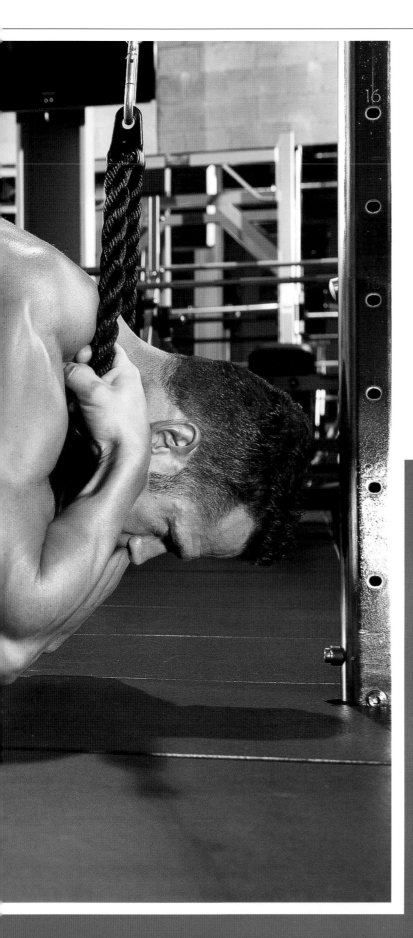

**OBLIQUE CRUNCH**
>> Lie on your side with your knees bent 90 degrees and touching each other. Start with your hands behind your head and your elbows back. Crunch straight up to the ceiling by contracting your oblique and abdominal muscles. Squeeze the obliques hard for a count or two, then lower back down.

**HANGING KNEE RAISE**
>> Hang from a pullup station using a wide grip and allowing your legs to hang straight down toward the floor, eyes facing forward. Contract your abs to raise your thighs to roughly parallel to the floor, bending your knees as you raise your legs. Lower slowly and repeat.

## WEEKS 3 & 4
Do each of the following exercises for 15 reps (or until failure) in giant-set fashion for 25 minutes:

*Hanging Knee Raise*
*Reverse Crunch*
*Crunch*
*Oblique Crunch*
*Oblique Crossover Crunch*
*Rope Crunch*

## WEEKS 5 & 6
Do each of the following exercises for 20 reps (or until failure) in giant-set fashion for 30 minutes:

*Hanging Knee Raise*
*Reverse Crunch*
*Double Crunch*
*Crunch*
*Oblique Crunch*
*Oblique Crossover Crunch*
*Rope Crunch*

# ABS DONE YOUR WAY

**With our fully customizable GrAB Bag program, you can finally get a ripped midsection with none of the boredom.**

Watching grass grow. Waiting for water to boil. Watching paint dry. These are just a few mind-numbing activites that are still more exciting than an ab workout filled with nothing but situps and crunches. And it's no wonder: You learned to do a situp in middle school and you were bored with crunches by the time you were a sophomore in college. What you need is an all-encompassing ab program that lets you choose from a variety of exercises. What you need is a GrAB Bag.

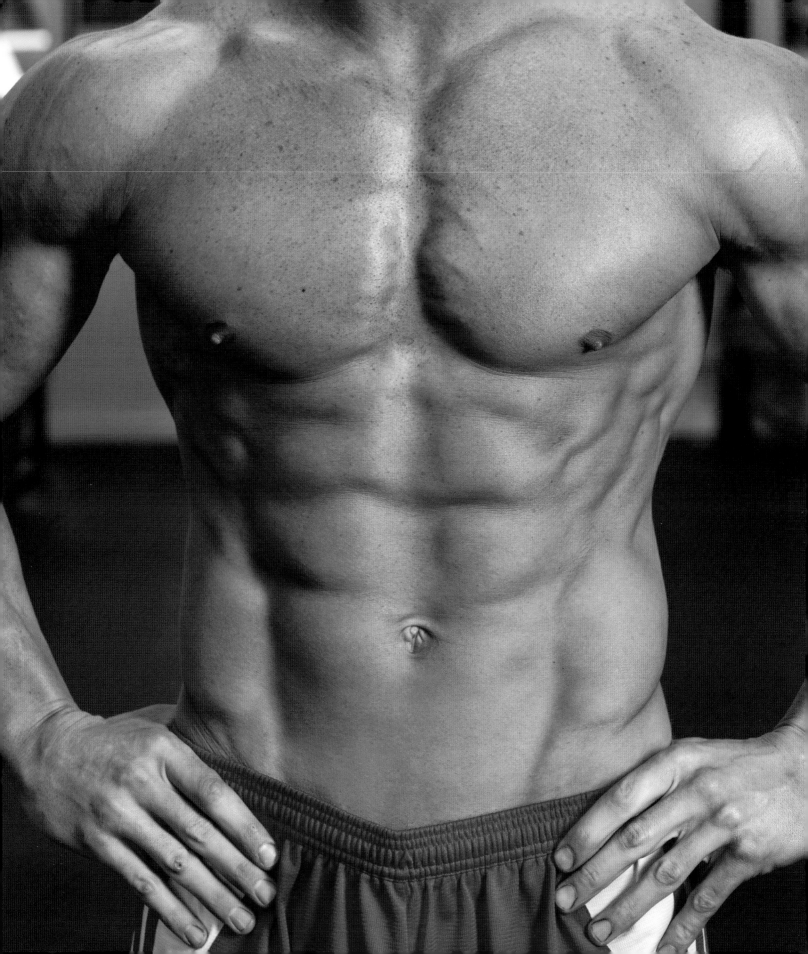

# BAG MAN

The GrAB Bag is a user-friendly method of choosing exercises that work all four abdominal muscles: the rectus abdominis (upper and lower portions), the internal and external obliques, and the transverse abdominis. Without question, the most effective ab program is one that targets every area. Additionally, the rep range is critical to the development of a strong and visible six-pack. Keeping your reps at 15–30 will help you maintain a flat and lean midsection while making your waist appear smaller.

The GrAB Bag program is simple: Each time you train abs, choose up to five exercises, one for each area (upper abs, lower abs, obliques, transverse abdominis). If you want to target a particular section with greater intensity, we've designed this program so you can do some one-stop shopping for your own personal top-of-the-line sixer.

Always hit your abs last in your workout. You shouldn't fatigue them before training other body parts, especially back or legs, because you want your core to be strong to help sustain the intra-abdominal pressure necessary to protect your spine.

# GRAB ABS

The main point of this program is to give you the abs you yearn for while staving off boredom, and customizing your routine helps you do just that. While most ab exercises hit more than one muscle, you can work a particular area by choosing specific exercises from the categories below.

Note: A higher rep range is designed to improve endurance and lean out, while the weighted versions, in the 8- to 12-rep range, build more thickness and size. Rest 30-120 seconds between sets, depending on the intensity and your overall goal. Decrease rest periods to enhance calorie-burning and intensity; increase them when performing weighted moves with the goal of hypertrophy. Finally, as you adapt to these exercises, increase the number of sets or add weight to standard body-weight-only exercises. The more you challenge yourself each week, the better your chances of crafting a hard, ripped midsection.

# À LA CARTE EXERCISE MENU

| UPPER ABS | CORE-SPECIFIC | LOWER ABS | COMBINATIONS | OBLIQUES |
|---|---|---|---|---|
| Crunch | Plank | Reverse Crunch | Double Crunch | Oblique Crunch |
| Weighted Crunch | Side Plank | Hip Thrust | Hanging Knee Raise/Twist | Bicycle |
| Lying Cable Crunch | Cable Woodchop | Scissor Kick | Decline Medicine-Ball Crunch/Twist/Throw | Crossover Crunch |
| Standing Cable Crunch | Wheel Roll-Out | Exercise-Ball Roll-In | Jackknife | Standing Oblique Cable Crunch |
| Decline Cable Situp | Dragon Flag | Reverse Crunch on Decline | Exercise Ball Transfer Crunch | Roman Chair Russian Twist |
| Roman Chair Weighted Situp | | Hanging Running in Place | | Lying Weighted Windshield Wiper |
| Supported Crunch | | Hanging Leg Raise | | Dumbbell Oblique Crunch |
| Exercise-Ball Crunch | | Hanging Knee Raise | | |
| Medicine-Ball Chop | | | | |

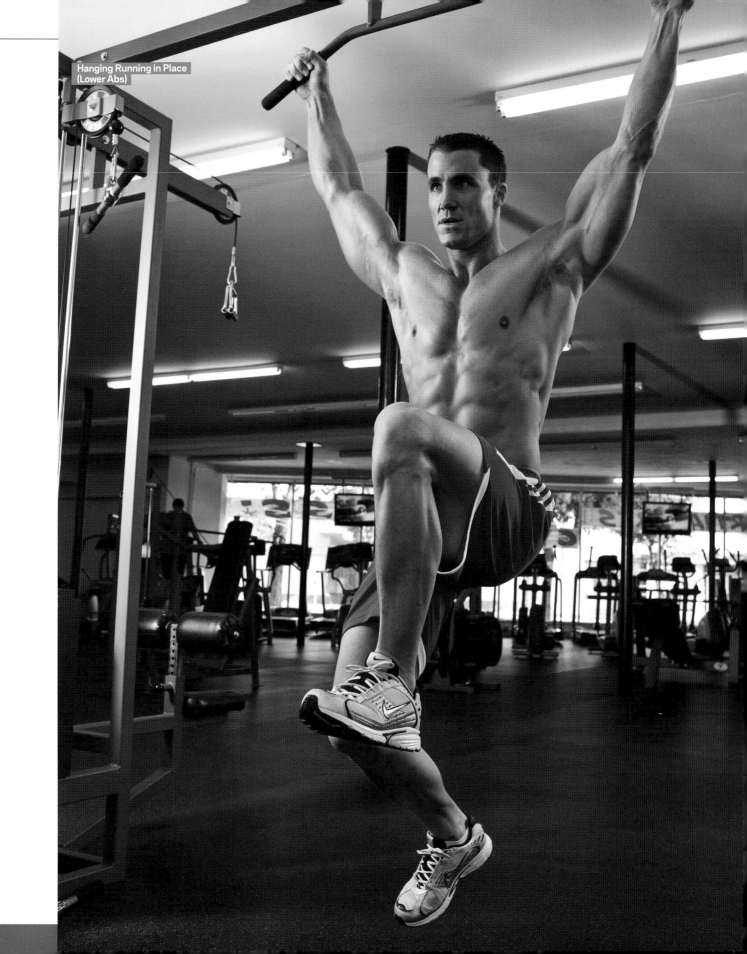

Hanging Running in Place
(Lower Abs)

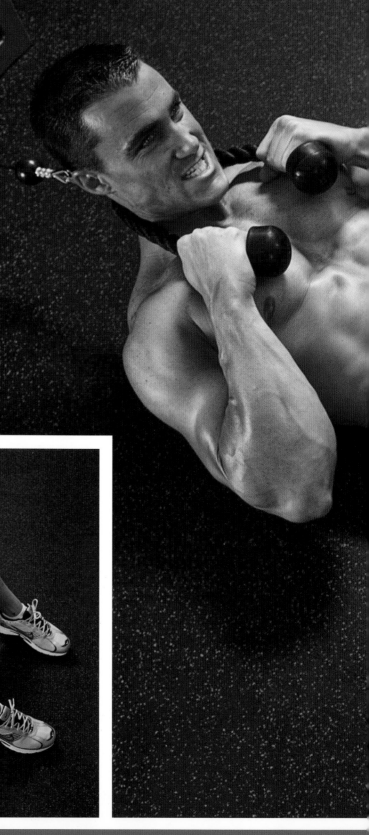

Lying Cable Crunch
(Upper Abs)

# CUSTOMIZE YOUR
# OVERALL
# ABS

Even though you can't completely isolate any one portion of the abdominals, you can involve a particular section to a greater extent through exercise selection. So to attack your abs with all sorts of moves means you're sure to cover the bases for a balanced midsection.

*1 Upper-Ab Exercise*
*1 Lower-Ab Exercise*
*1 Obliques Exercise*
*1 Core-Specific Exercise*
*1 Combination Exercise*

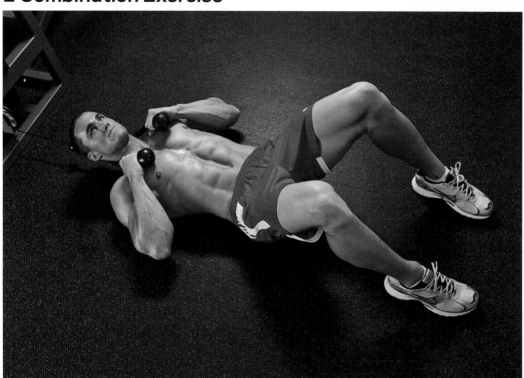

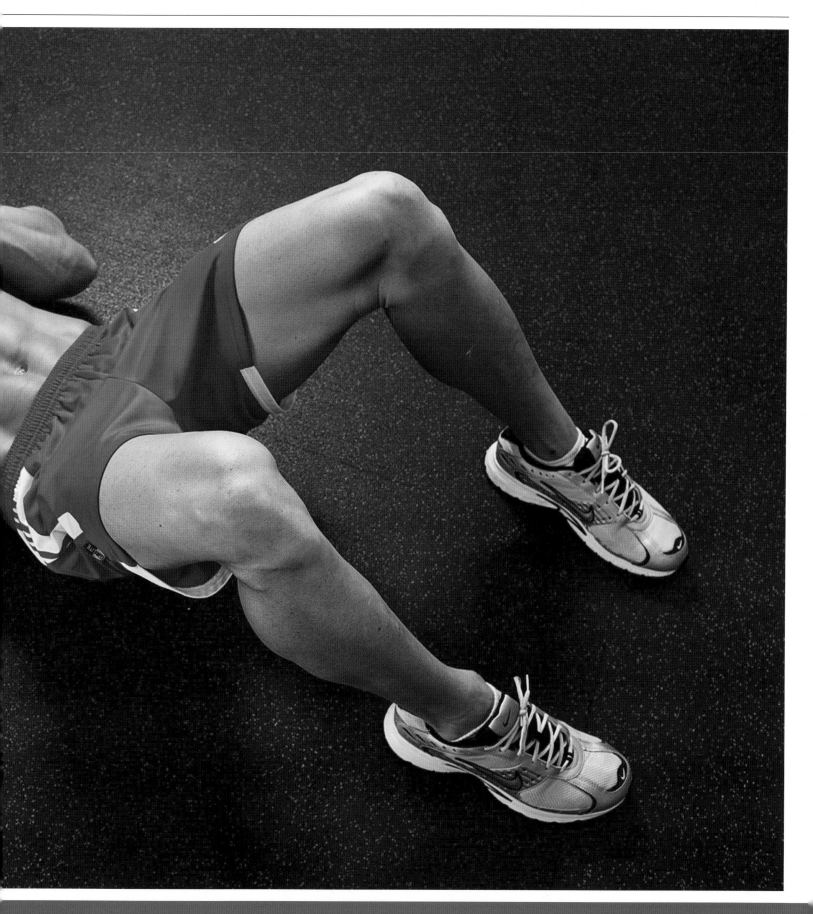

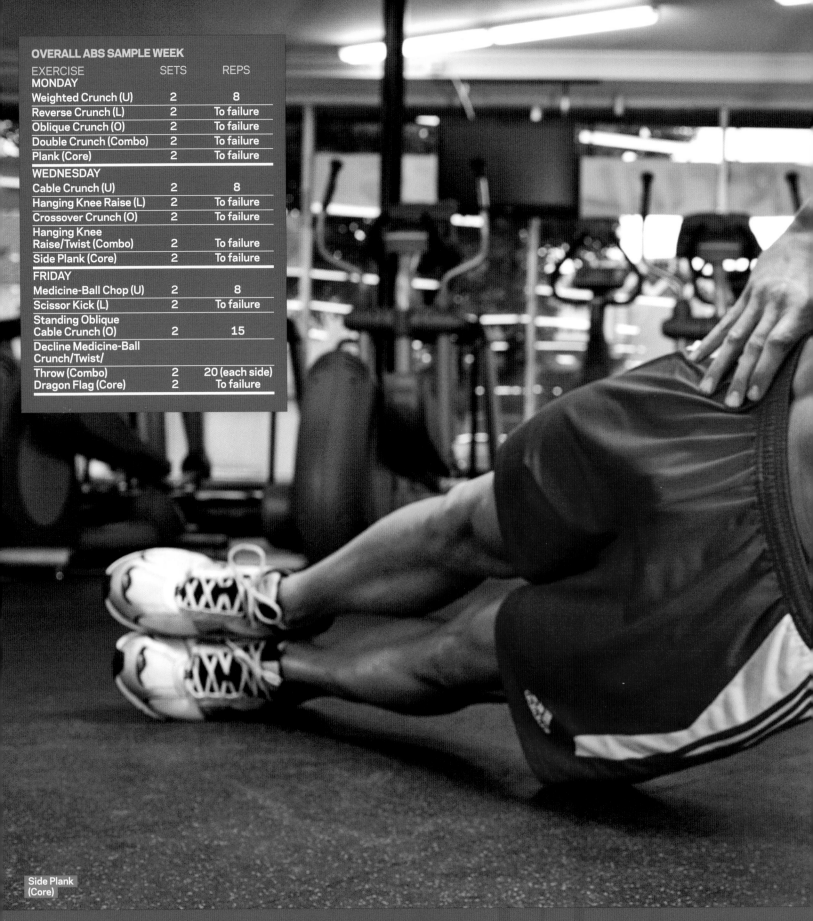

## OVERALL ABS SAMPLE WEEK

| EXERCISE | SETS | REPS |
|---|---|---|
| **MONDAY** | | |
| Weighted Crunch (U) | 2 | 8 |
| Reverse Crunch (L) | 2 | To failure |
| Oblique Crunch (O) | 2 | To failure |
| Double Crunch (Combo) | 2 | To failure |
| Plank (Core) | 2 | To failure |
| **WEDNESDAY** | | |
| Cable Crunch (U) | 2 | 8 |
| Hanging Knee Raise (L) | 2 | To failure |
| Crossover Crunch (O) | 2 | To failure |
| Hanging Knee Raise/Twist (Combo) | 2 | To failure |
| Side Plank (Core) | 2 | To failure |
| **FRIDAY** | | |
| Medicine-Ball Chop (U) | 2 | 8 |
| Scissor Kick (L) | 2 | To failure |
| Standing Oblique Cable Crunch (O) | 2 | 15 |
| Decline Medicine-Ball Crunch/Twist/ Throw (Combo) | 2 | 20 (each side) |
| Dragon Flag (Core) | 2 | To failure |

Side Plank (Core)

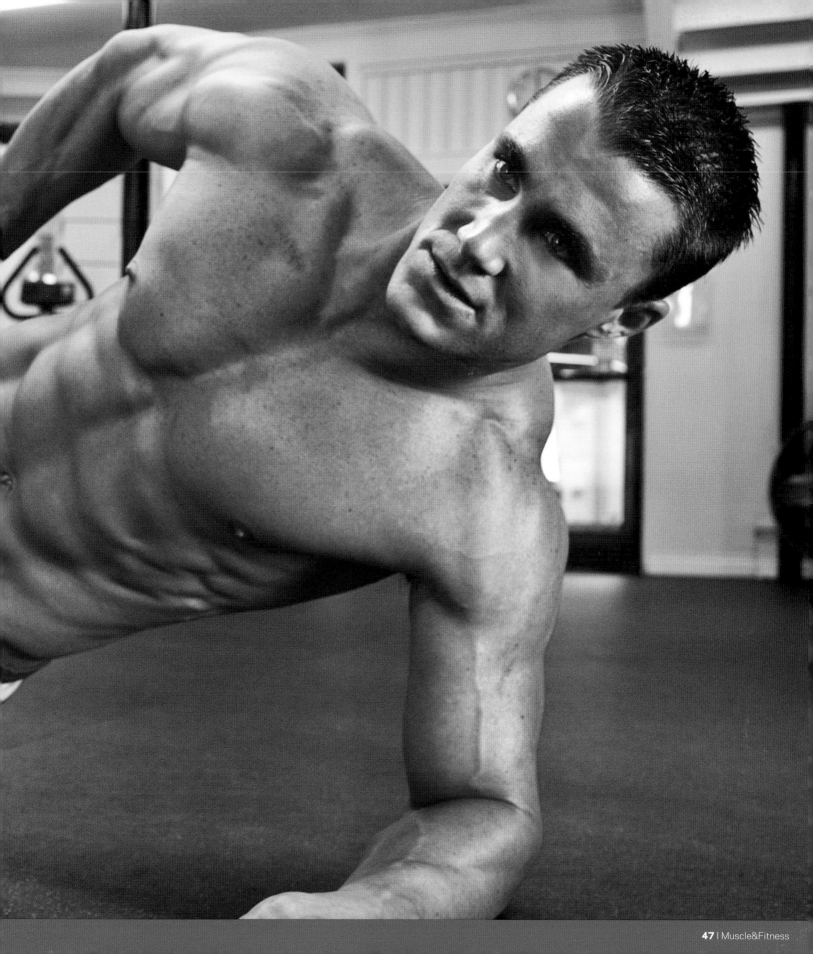

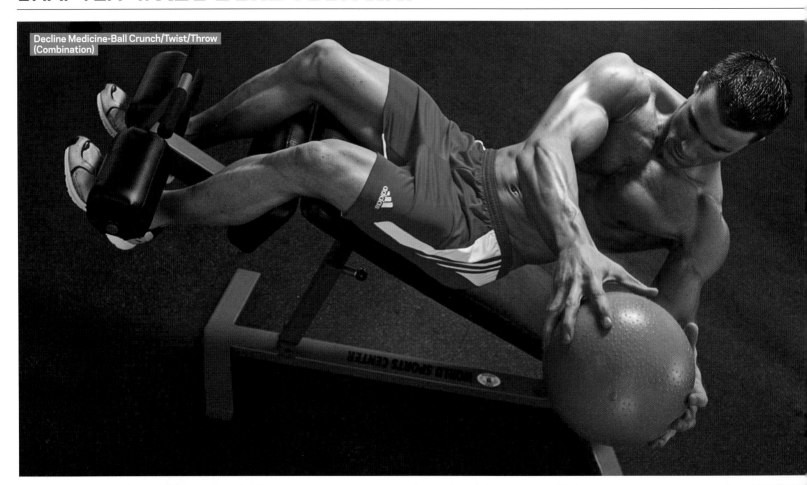

Decline Medicine-Ball Crunch/Twist/Throw (Combination)

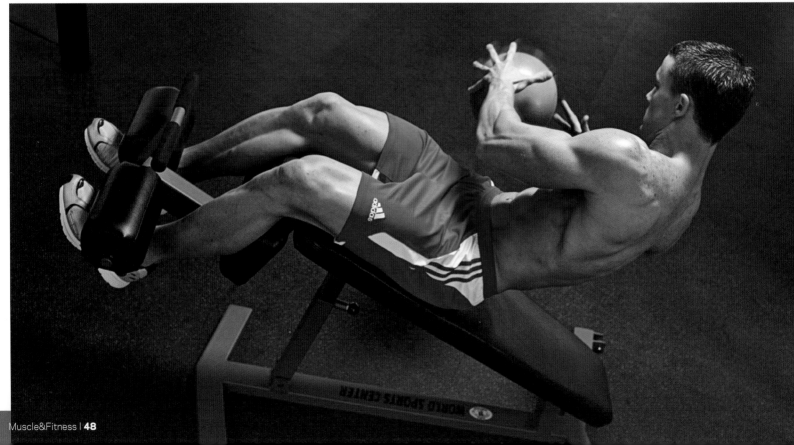

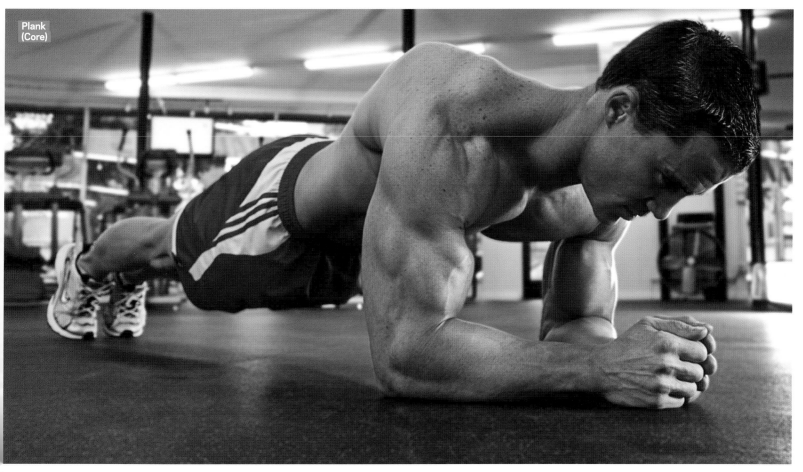

Plank
(Core)

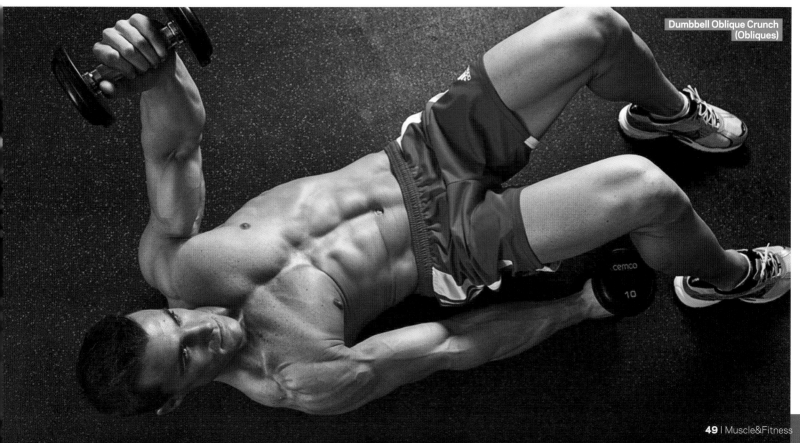

Dumbbell Oblique Crunch
(Obliques)

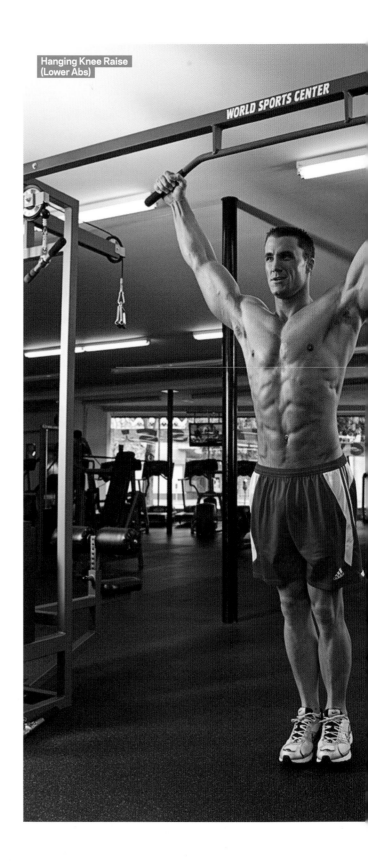

Hanging Knee Raise
(Lower Abs)

# CUSTOMIZE YOUR
# LOWER ABS

For many a weightlifter, the lower abs are the weakest of the ab muscles. The key to targeting them is to bring your legs toward your torso. If your lower abs are a weakness, try doing them first in your ab routine.

## 1 Upper-Ab Exercise
## 3 Lower-Ab Exercises
## 1 Obliques Exercise

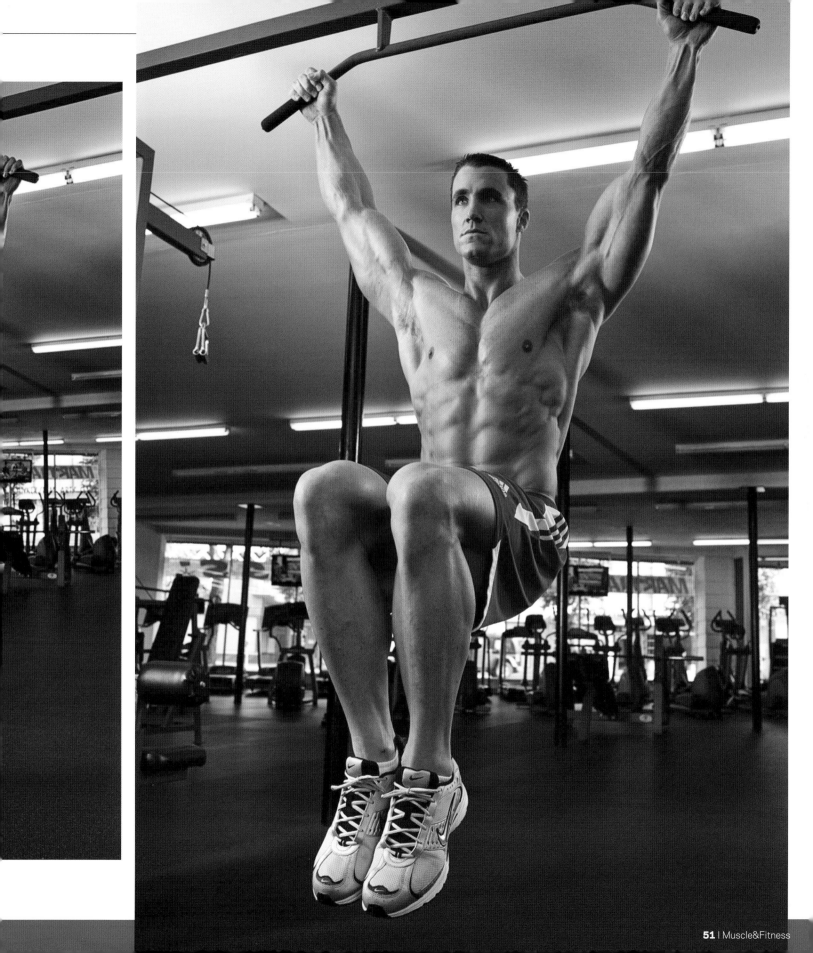

## LOWER ABS SAMPLE WEEK

| EXERCISE | SETS | REPS |
|---|---|---|
| **MONDAY** | | |
| Weighted Crunch (U) | 2 | 10 |
| Hanging Knee Raise (L) | 2 | To failure |
| Hip Thrust (L) | 2 | To failure |
| Reverse Crunch (L) | 2 | To failure |
| Oblique Crunch (O) | 2 | To failure |
| **WEDNESDAY** | | |
| Supported Crunch (U) | 2 | To failure |
| Hanging Leg Raise (L) | 2 | To failure |
| Scissor Kick (L) | 2 | To failure |
| Reverse Crunch (L) | 2 | To failure |
| Crossover Crunch (O) | 2 | To failure |
| **FRIDAY** | | |
| Weighted Crunch (U) | 2 | 10 |
| Exercise-Ball Roll-In (L) | 2 | 10 |
| Hanging Running in Place (L) | 2 | To failure |
| Reverse Crunch on Decline (L) | 2 | To failure |
| Standing Oblique Cable Crunch (O) | 2 | 15 |

Scissor Kick
(Lower Abs)

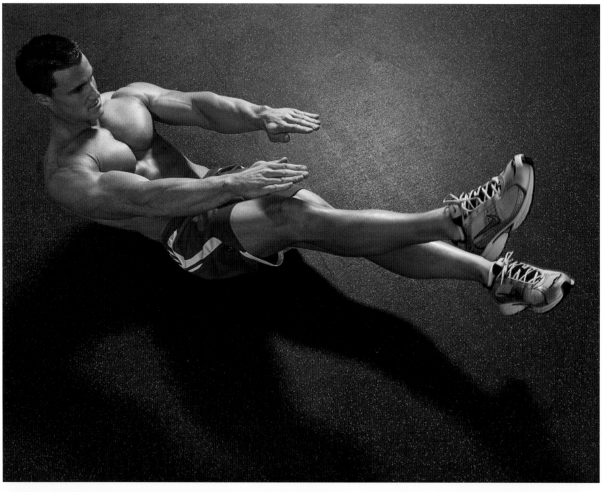

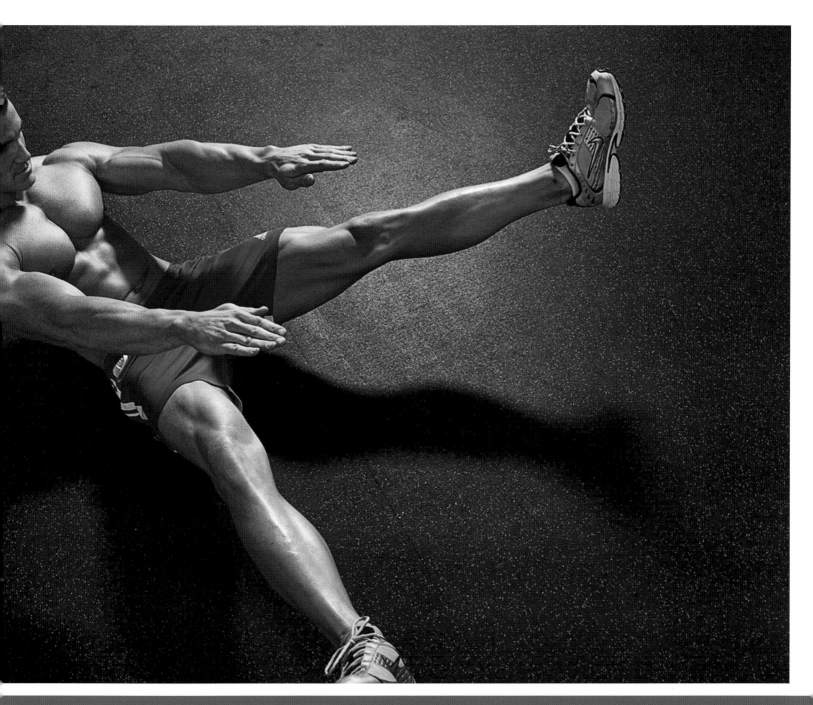

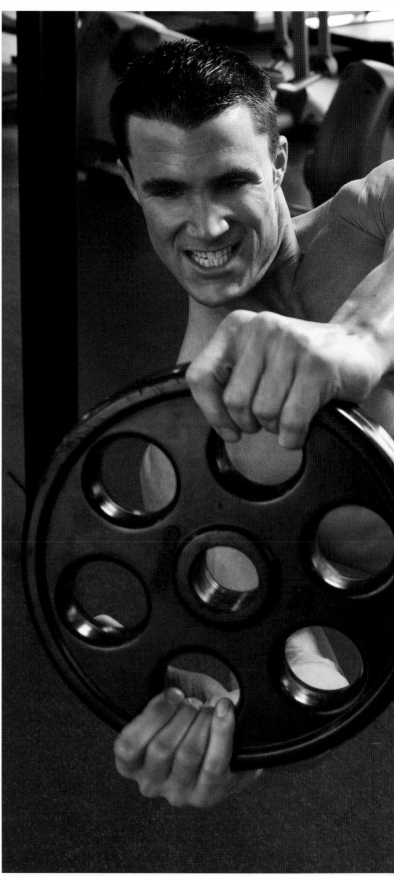

# CUSTOMIZE YOUR
# UPPER ABS

The upper abs are arguably your strongest "ab assets." Anytime you bring your torso toward your legs, you target the upper abs. If you want your abs to show deeper cuts, adding weight to your favorite moves is your best bet.

*2 Upper-Ab Exercises*
*1 Lower-Ab Exercise*
*1 Core-Specific Exercise*
*1 Combination Exercise*

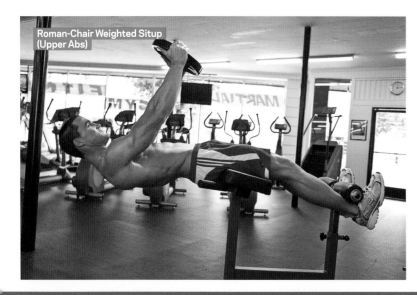

Roman-Chair Weighted Situp
(Upper Abs)

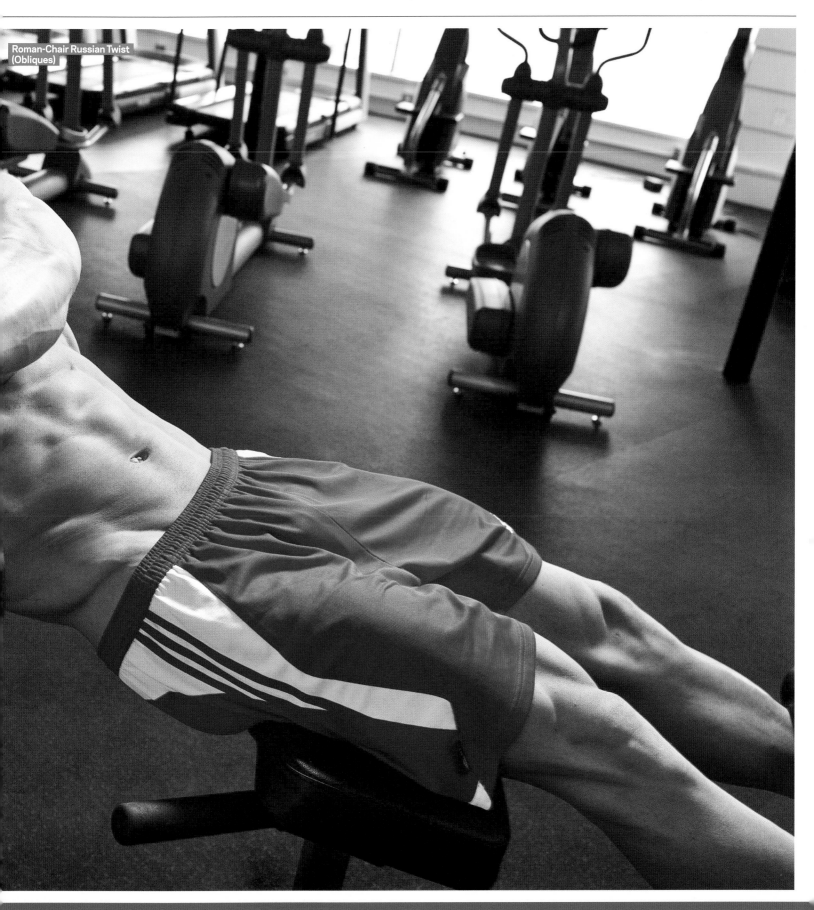

Roman-Chair Russian Twist
(Obliques)

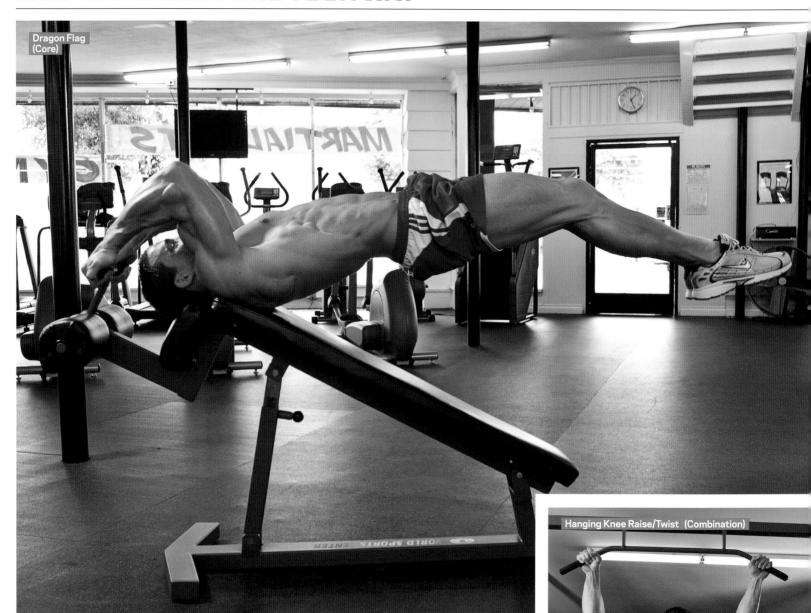

Dragon Flag (Core)

Hanging Knee Raise/Twist (Combination)

**UPPER ABS SAMPLE WEEK**

| EXERCISE | SETS | REPS |
|---|---|---|
| **MONDAY/THURSDAY** | | |
| Cable Crunch (U) | 2 | 8 |
| Roman Chair Weighted Situp (U) | 2 | 25 |
| Reverse Crunch (L) | 2 | To failure |
| Plank (Core) | 2 | To failure |
| Double Crunch (Combo) | 2 | To failure |
| **TUESDAY/FRIDAY** | | |
| Crunch (U) | 2 | To failure |
| Medicine-Ball Chop (U) | 2 | 20 |
| Hanging Knee Raise (L) | 2 | To failure |
| Dragon Flag (Core) | 2 | To failure |
| Hanging Knee Raise/Twist (Combo) | 1 | To failure |

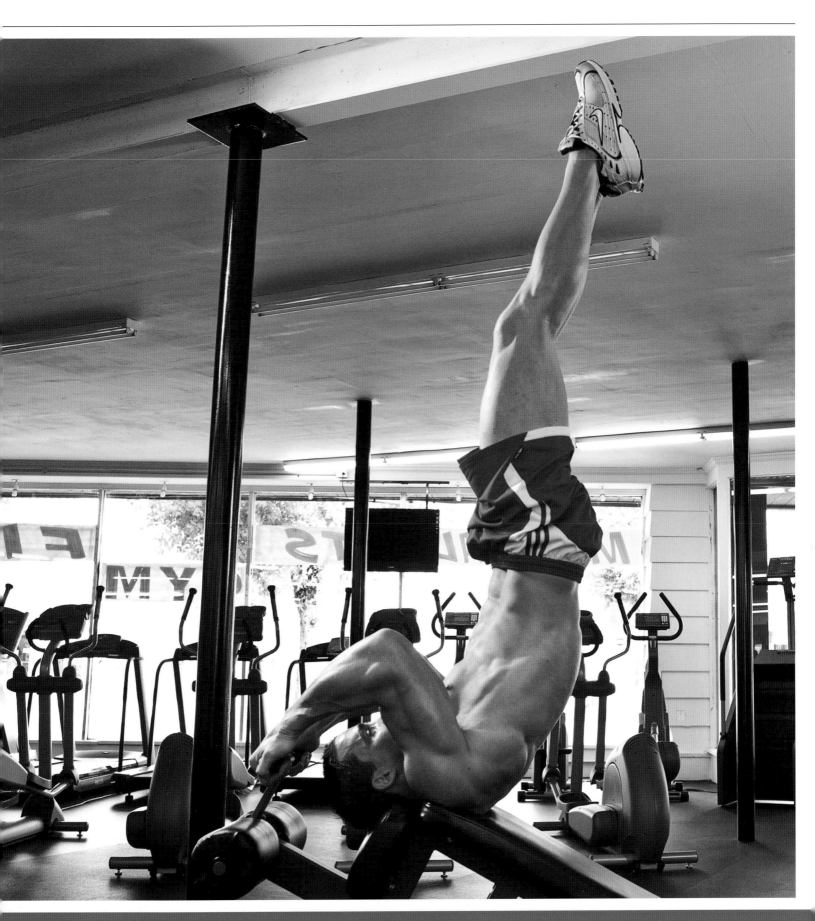

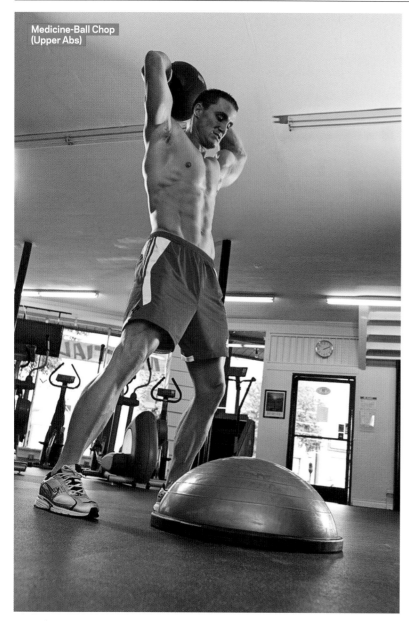

Medicine-Ball Chop (Upper Abs)

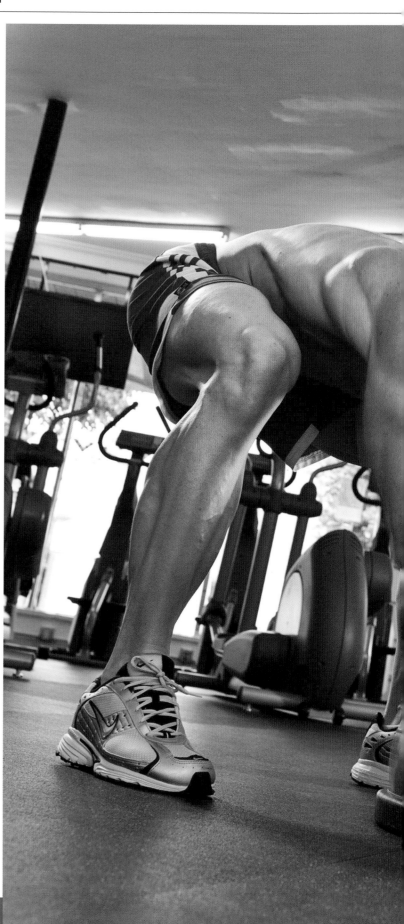

# CUSTOMIZE YOUR
# OBLIQUES

Helping complete the abdominal package are the internal and external obliques, which are responsible for trunk rotation and lateral flexion of the torso. Strong obliques are also integral to athletic performance. If you've neglected your obliques, the imbalance will be detected when you begin these exercises.

*1 Upper-Ab Exercise*
*1 Lower-Ab Exercise*
*2 Obliques Exercises*
*1 Core-Specific Exercise*

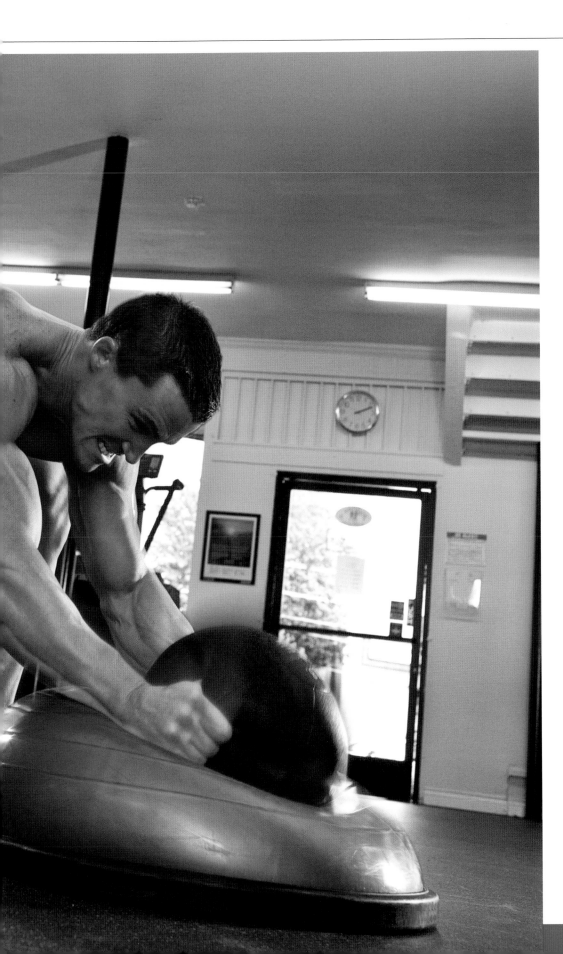

# Diet Done Your Way

**We've given you the workout that'll make your abs pop. Now here's the diet to make your belly fat drop.**

Similar to the GrAB Bag training plan, the GrAB Bag diet plan allows you to select the meals you want so you can piece together your own nutritional program.

The meal plan goes like this: Pick one meal card each from the breakfast bag, morning snack bag, lunch bag, afternoon snack bag, dinner bag, and before-bed snack bag; and on workout days add a meal from the pre-workout and post-workout bags. Your daily totals will be 2,200–2,500 calories, 240–260 grams of protein, 140–180 grams of carbs and 60–90 grams of fat. That's perfect for those who weigh 160–200 pounds.

For a 180-pound guy, for example, a workout day delivers 12–14 calories, 1.25–1.5 grams of protein, just under 1 gram of carbs and 0.25–0.5 gram of fat per pound of body weight. On rest days, skip the pre- and post-workout meals. Then you'll net about 2,000 calories or about 11 calories per pound, including 200 grams of protein and about 100 grams of carbs per day.

Be sure to allow two or three hours between meals. While you should eat breakfast immediately after waking, all other meals should follow the 30-minute rule: Eat pre- and post-workout meals within 30 minutes of exercising, and take your before-bed snack 30 minutes before you hit the sack. We also suggest that every 7–10 days you throw in a cheat meal in which you triple your carbs. This diet plan will help you melt off fat, but sticking with it for too long could stall your metabolism. A cheat day will help your body maintain high levels of leptin, which decreases hunger and speeds up your metabolic rate. Follow this plan and you'll be on your way to ripped abs in about eight weeks.

## MORNING SNACK BAG

**OPTION 1**
1 cup **low-fat cottage cheese**
1 cup **sliced pineapple**

**Option 2**
1 scoop **whey protein**
1 cup **oatmeal**

**OPTION 3**
4–6 oz **low-fat plain yogurt**
1 tbsp **peanut butter**

**OPTION 4**
1 cup **low-fat cottage cheese**
6 **whole-wheat crackers** +
1 tbsp **peanut butter**

**OPTION 5**
*Turkey rolls:*
2 slices **turkey deli meat**
2 slices **low-fat American cheese**
¼ **avocado**

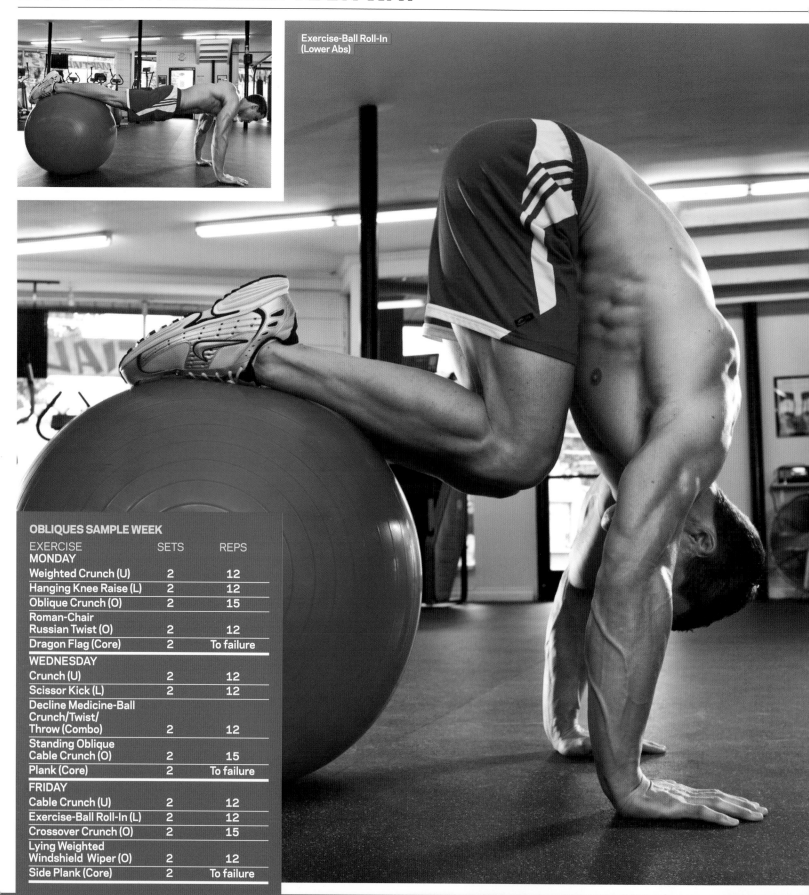

Exercise-Ball Roll-In
(Lower Abs)

| OBLIQUES SAMPLE WEEK | | |
|---|---|---|
| EXERCISE | SETS | REPS |
| **MONDAY** | | |
| Weighted Crunch (U) | 2 | 12 |
| Hanging Knee Raise (L) | 2 | 12 |
| Oblique Crunch (O) | 2 | 15 |
| Roman-Chair Russian Twist (O) | 2 | 12 |
| Dragon Flag (Core) | 2 | To failure |
| **WEDNESDAY** | | |
| Crunch (U) | 2 | 12 |
| Scissor Kick (L) | 2 | 12 |
| Decline Medicine-Ball Crunch/Twist/ Throw (Combo) | 2 | 12 |
| Standing Oblique Cable Crunch (O) | 2 | 15 |
| Plank (Core) | 2 | To failure |
| **FRIDAY** | | |
| Cable Crunch (U) | 2 | 12 |
| Exercise-Ball Roll-In (L) | 2 | 12 |
| Crossover Crunch (O) | 2 | 15 |
| Lying Weighted Windshield Wiper (O) | 2 | 12 |
| Side Plank (Core) | 2 | To failure |

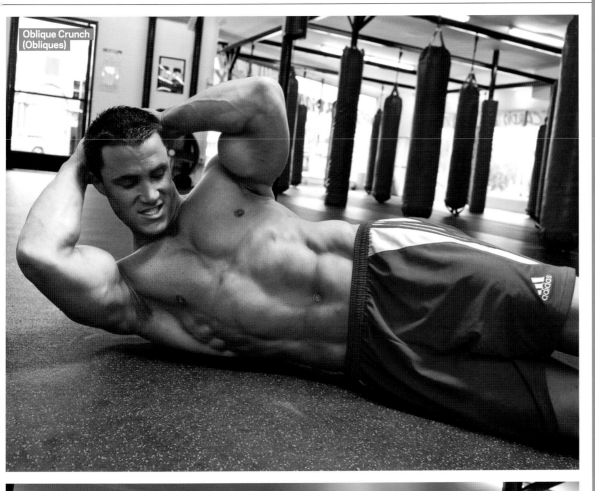

Oblique Crunch
(Obliques)

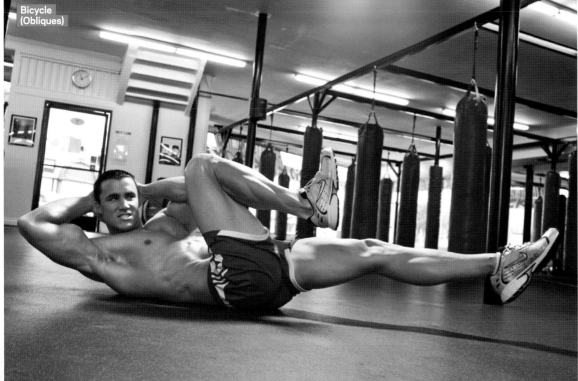

Bicycle
(Obliques)

1 tbsp **light mayo**
*Layer one slice cheese on one slice turkey, spread mayo on cheese, layer on avocado; roll meat and cheese around avocado.*

**BREAKFAST BAG**

OPTION 1
3 whole eggs + 3 egg whites
½ cup **Raisin Bran** +
½ cup **low-fat milk**

OPTION 2
2 scoops **whey protein**
1 medium **banana**

OPTION 3
3 whole eggs + 3 egg whites
1 cup **oatmeal**

OPTION 4
1 *Western Bagel's Perfect 10 Bagel Healthy Grain* +
1 tbsp *light cream cheese*
1 cup **low-fat milk**

OPTION 5
3 whole **eggs**
1 slice **low-fat American cheese**
3 slices **Jennie-O Extra Lean Turkey Bacon**
1 cup **oatmeal**

**LUNCH BAG**

OPTION 1
4 slices **roast beef** +
2 slices **whole-wheat bread**
1 cup **broccoli**

OPTION 2
1 can **albacore tuna** +
2 slices **whole-wheat bread** +
1 tbsp **fat-free mayo**

OPTION 3
4 oz **95% lean ground beef** +
1 slice **low-fat American cheese** +
1 **whole-wheat hamburger bun**

OPTION 4
1 can **albacore tuna** +
1 tbsp **light mayo** +
1 large **whole-wheat pita pocket**

OPTION 5
½ can (3 oz) **albacore tuna**
½ cup **low-fat cottage cheese**
2 cups **mixed green salad** +
2 tbsp **olive oil/vinegar dressing**
1 cup **blueberries**

**AFTERNOON SNACK BAG**

OPTION 1
1 cup **low-fat cottage cheese** +
2 tbsp **salsa**

OPTION 2
2 sticks **light mozzarella string cheese**

OPTION 3
2 oz **beef jerky**

OPTION 4
1 oz **fat-free cheese (Swiss, cheddar, or Monterey Jack)**
2 slices **turkey deli meat**
1 oz **mixed nuts**

OPTION 5
4 oz **shrimp** +
1 tbsp **seafood cocktail sauce**

**DINNER BAG**

OPTION 1
8 oz **top sirloin**
1 cup **broccoli**
2 cups **mixed green salad** +
2 tbsp **olive oil/vinegar dressing**

OPTION 2
9 oz **tilapia**
10 **asparagus spears**

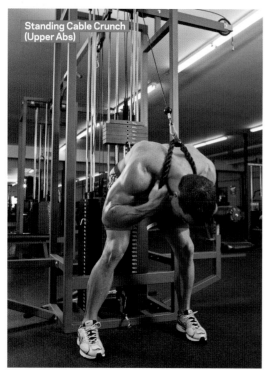

Standing Cable Crunch
(Upper Abs)

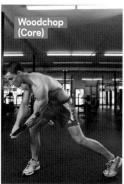

Woodchop
(Core)

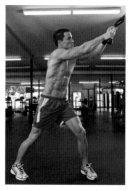

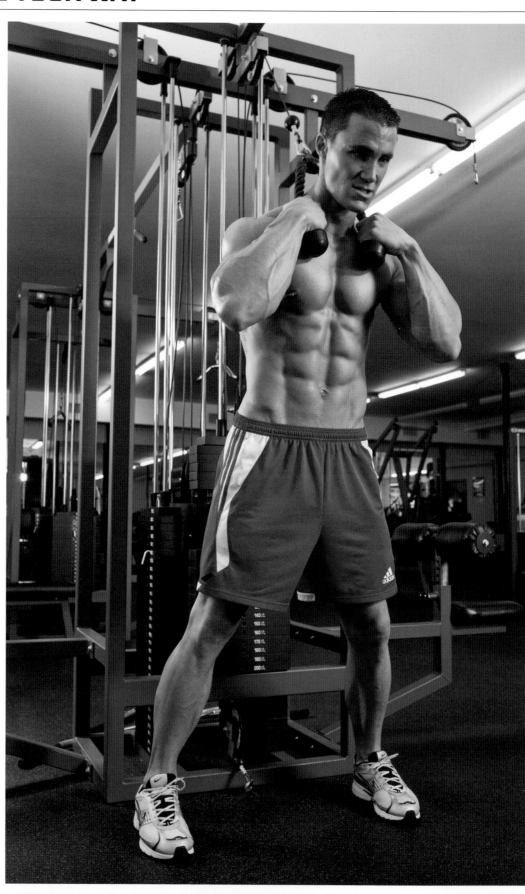

# CUSTOMIZE YOUR CORE

While all of these muscles make up the overall core, here we're talking about the innermost abdominal muscles. Think of the transverse abdominis as an internal weight belt, helping provide stability to your spine by producing intra-abdominal pressure. This pressure, much like that provided by a weight belt, helps keep the spine in safe alignment during bentover and squatting moves.

*1 Upper-Ab Exercise*
*1 Lower-Ab Exercise*
*2 Core-Specific Exercises*

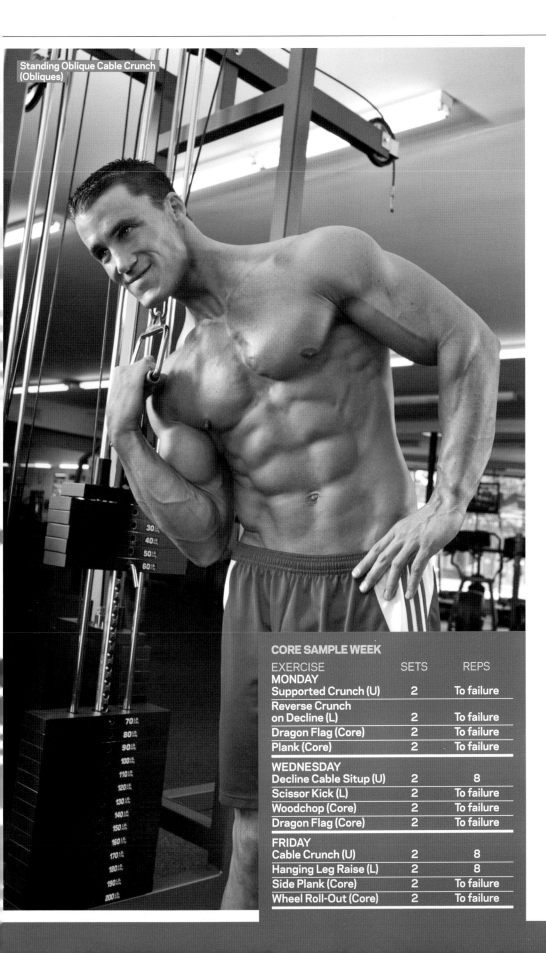

Standing Oblique Cable Crunch (Obliques)

**CORE SAMPLE WEEK**

| EXERCISE | SETS | REPS |
|---|---|---|
| **MONDAY** | | |
| Supported Crunch (U) | 2 | To failure |
| Reverse Crunch on Decline (L) | 2 | To failure |
| Dragon Flag (Core) | 2 | To failure |
| Plank (Core) | 2 | To failure |
| **WEDNESDAY** | | |
| Decline Cable Situp (U) | 2 | 8 |
| Scissor Kick (L) | 2 | To failure |
| Woodchop (Core) | 2 | To failure |
| Dragon Flag (Core) | 2 | To failure |
| **FRIDAY** | | |
| Cable Crunch (U) | 2 | 8 |
| Hanging Leg Raise (L) | 2 | 8 |
| Side Plank (Core) | 2 | To failure |
| Wheel Roll-Out (Core) | 2 | To failure |

2 cups **mixed green salad** +
2 tbsp **olive oil/vinegar dressing**
**OPTION 3**
8 oz **chicken breast**
1 cup **sliced zucchini**
2 cups **green salad** +
2 tbsp **olive oil/vinegar dressing**
**OPTION 4**
9 oz **farmed Atlantic salmon**
½ cup **mixed frozen veggies**
2 cups **mixed green salad** +
2 tbsp **olive oil/vinegar dressing**
**OPTION 5**
*Chili Con Carne:*
6 oz **lean ground beef**
3.5 oz **canned diced tomatoes with chiles**
¼ **medium onion**
*Brown beef in pan; add tomatoes, chopped onion, 1/2 tsp ground cumin, 1 tsp chili powder, and salt and pepper to taste.*

**BEFORE-BED SNACK BAG**
**OPTION 1**
1 cup **low-fat cottage cheese** +
2 tbsp **roasted flaxseeds**
**OPTION 2**
1 scoop **casein protein**
1 tbsp **peanut butter**
**OPTION 3**
1 cup **low-fat cottage cheese**
1 tbsp **peanut butter**
**OPTION 4**
2 oz **fat-free cheese (Swiss, cheddar, or Monterey Jack)**
2 medium **celery stalks** +
1 tbsp **peanut butter**
**OPTION 5**
1 scoop **casein protein** +
1 tbsp **flaxseed oil**

**PRE-WORKOUT BAG**
**OPTION 1**
1 scoop **whey protein**
**OPTION 2**
1 scoop **soy protein**
**OPTION 3**
½ scoop **whey** +
½ scoop **soy protein**
**OPTION 4**
1 scoop **mixed protein powder (whey, casein, milk, soy, or egg protein)**
**OPTION 5**
Low-carb ready-to-drink protein shake

**POST-WORKOUT BAG**
**OPTION 1**
1 scoop **whey protein** +
1 scoop **casein protein**
½ medium plain **bagel** + 1 tbsp **jelly**
**OPTION 2**
1 scoop **whey protein** +
1 scoop **casein protein**
1 large slice **angel food cake**
**OPTION 3**
1 scoop **whey protein** + 1 scoop **casein protein** + 20 oz **Gatorade**
**OPTION 4**
1 scoop **whey protein** +
1 scoop **casein protein**
40 **jelly beans**
**OPTION 5**
1 scoop **whey protein** + 1 scoop **casein protein** + 1 scoop **Vitargo**
*NOTE: Mix all protein powders according to directions on the label.*

# CHAPTER 5

# WORKING ALL THE ANGLES

**Basic crunching isn't enough. For strong, attractive and totally functional abs you have to curl, bend, and twist.**

When it comes to sculpting a lean, chiseled six-pack, most guys believe it takes the right mix of exercises to get the job done. But the key to maximum results in minimal time may not be so much the moves you pick, but rather picking the right way to move.

First, here's some simple science: Whenever you use your abs, you're moving your body through one of three distinct planes of motion: sagittal, where you curl your torso or legs toward the other; frontal, where you bend side to side; and transverse, where you twist at the waist.

There's a reason this is important. "The more planes of motion you use to train a muscle, the more fibers you engage and the more adept it becomes at handling your demands," says Audrey Lynn Millar, Ph.D., P.T., professor of physical therapy at Andrews University (Berrien Springs, Michigan). "Most people choose sagittal-based exercises like crunches that train their midsections through only a single plane of motion," she explains. To make matters worse, "many common weight-training exercises such as squats, lunges, and presses isometrically contract the midsection through a sagittal plane of motion as well," Millar says. That means if you're not training your core through all three planes of motion in each workout, you're probably overworking certain muscle fibers and underutilizing others, leaving you more susceptible to injury and less likely to develop the washboard abs you're striving for.

Leaving no angle untrained guarantees you'll also see noticeable gains in other muscles. "Anytime you load weight above your waist—whether it's a bar across your back or dumbbells held in front of you—you're placing stress on your core musculature," says Rett Larson, C.S.C.S., U.S.A.W. Level 1, director of coaching at Velocity Sports Performance. "If your midsection isn't equally strong through all three planes, it may have a harder time handling the load, which can minimize the effectiveness of the exercise. An imbalanced core can also compromise your ability to properly perform Olympic lifts, plyometric exercises and other explosive-type movements that can vastly improve power, size, and strength."

Instead of focusing on specific areas of the muscle, the key to developing impressive abs—aesthetically and functionally—is choosing exercises that make you curl, bend, and twist at the waist all in the same workout. This routine lets you select your own exercises to thoroughly engage your midsection. Whichever moves you pick, you'll create a program that hits your abs from several angles to build a strong, flat midsection that works hard and, more important, looks even harder.

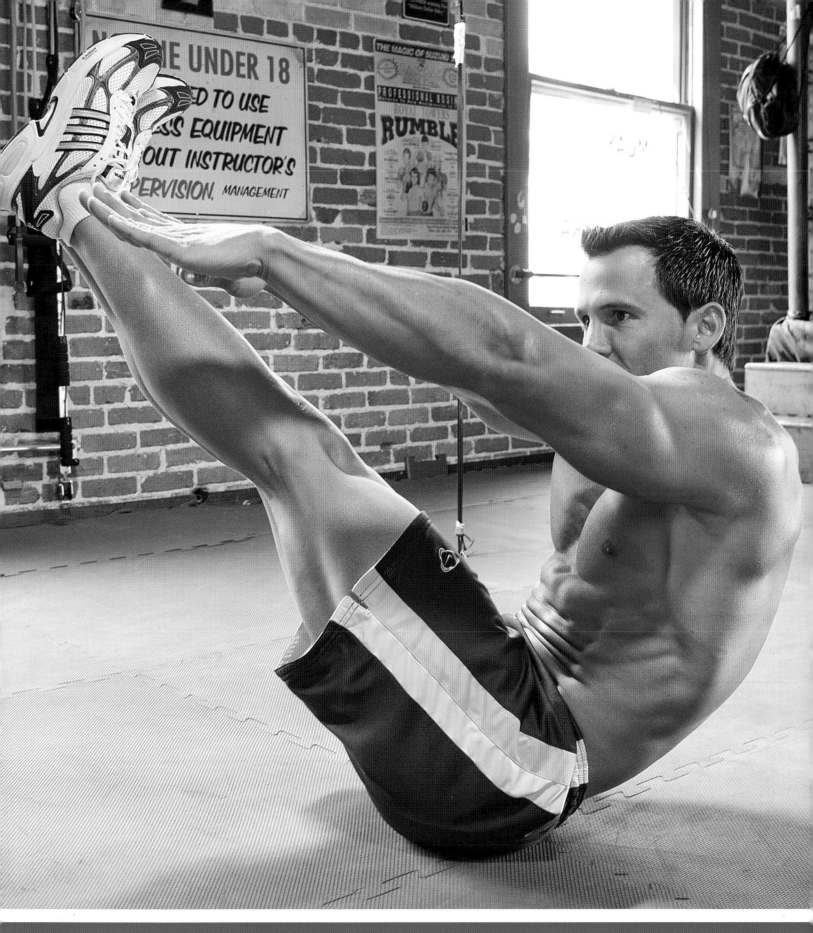

# WORKOUT RULES

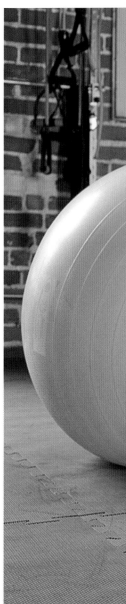

Pick one exercise each from "Curl It," "Twist It," and "Bend It." Do the first move for as many repetitions as possible, then move immediately to the second and third exercises, performing as many reps of each as you can. (If you select a move that uses added weight, choose a resistance that lets you get 20–25 reps while you're learning the exercise.) Once you finish all three exercises, rest for 30 seconds, then repeat the cycle twice more for a total of nine sets. Swap out your moves every two or three workouts. Once you're used to the exercises, switch up the weight you use so you can get 20–25 reps per set in some workouts, 12–20 reps in others, and even 8–10 reps per set in still other workouts.

## CURL IT EXERCISES

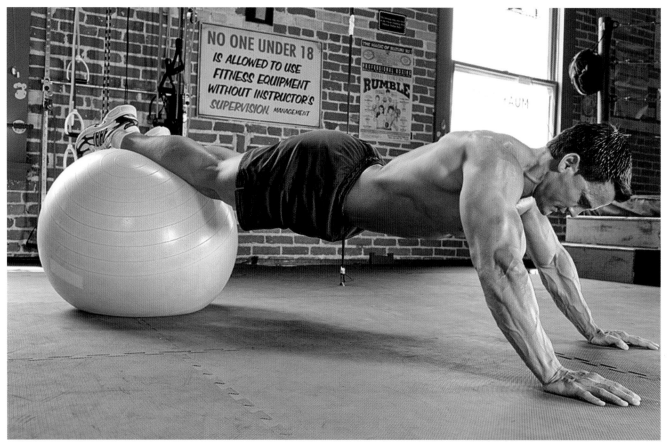

**EXERCISE-BALL KNEE TUCK**
Get into a push-up position with your feet up on an exercise ball. Maintaining a straight line from head to toes, slowly draw your knees toward your chest, rolling the ball toward you. Keep your hips down. Pause, then extend your legs, rolling the ball back even farther so your hands are 3–4 inches in front of your shoulders.

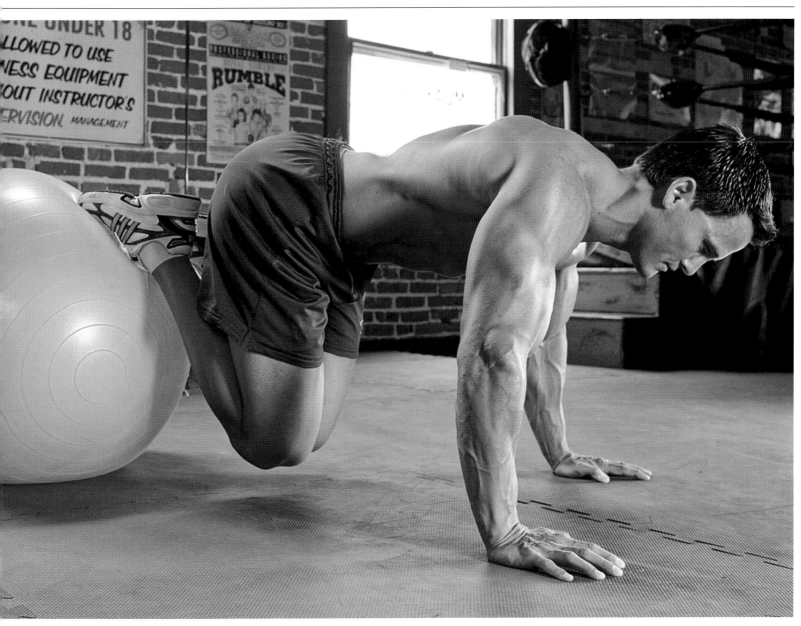

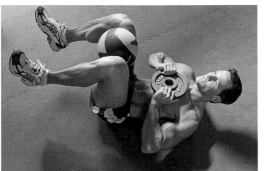

### WEIGHTED DOUBLE CRUNCH
Lie faceup with your knees bent and feet flat on the floor. Place a light medicine ball between your knees and grasp a weight plate (8–10 pounds to start) with both hands at your chest. Draw your knees toward your chest while simultaneously curling your shoulders off the floor. Pause, then lower back to the start.

### DOUBLE CRUNCH
Lie faceup with your knees bent and feet flat on the floor. Touch your fingers lightly to the sides of your head, pointing your elbows toward your knees. Curl your shoulders and upper back off the floor while simultaneously raising your knees. Pause, then lower back to the start.

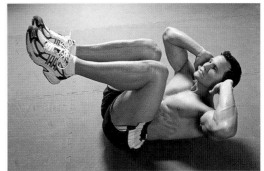

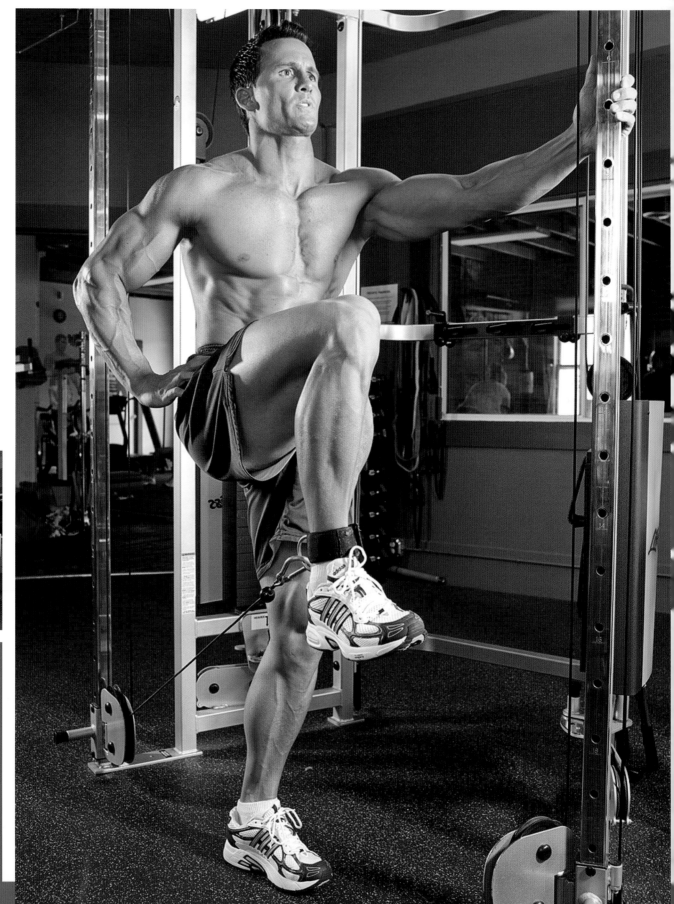

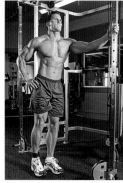

**STANDING CABLE KNEE RAISE**
Stand erect facing away from a low-pulley cable station and attach an ankle strap to your right leg. Grasp the tower for support. Keeping your back straight, slowly raise your right knee as high as you can. Pause, then lower back to the start. Repeat for reps, then switch sides.

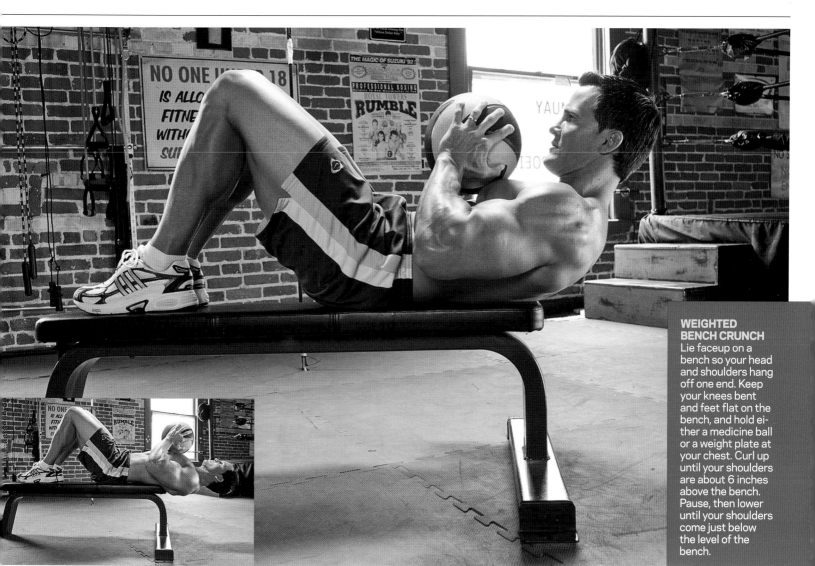

## WEIGHTED BENCH CRUNCH

Lie faceup on a bench so your head and shoulders hang off one end. Keep your knees bent and feet flat on the bench, and hold either a medicine ball or a weight plate at your chest. Curl up until your shoulders are about 6 inches above the bench. Pause, then lower until your shoulders come just below the level of the bench.

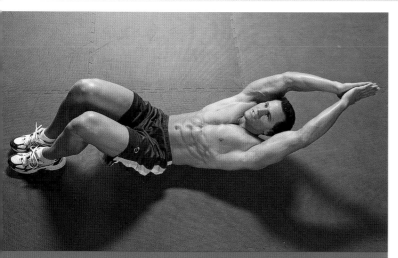

## OVERHEAD CRUNCH

Lie faceup with your knees bent, feet flat on the floor and arms extended overhead with your hands together. Keeping your arms straight and alongside your head, curl up to raise your shoulders off the floor. Pause, then lower back to the start.

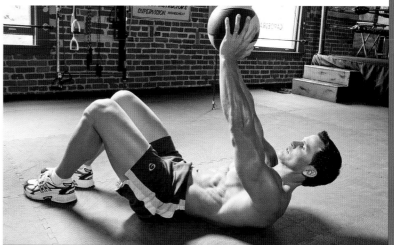

## ELEVATED BALL CRUNCH

Lie faceup with your knees bent and feet flat on the floor. Grasp a medicine ball with both hands and extend your arms to raise it over your chest. Curl up until your shoulders and upper back come off the floor. Pause, then lower back to the start. Repeat for reps.

# TWIST EXERCISES

## WEIGHTED TWIST/CRUNCH
Lie faceup with your knees bent and feet flat on the floor. Grasp a lightweight plate with both hands and extend your arms toward your knees. Slowly curl your torso off the floor and twist to the right, bringing the weight plate outside your right knee. Lower back down and alternate sides for reps.

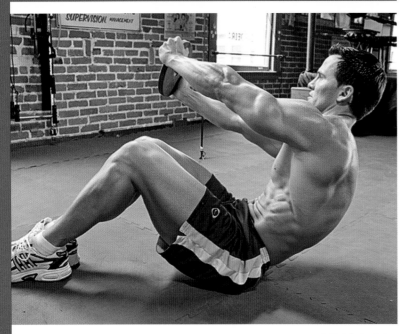

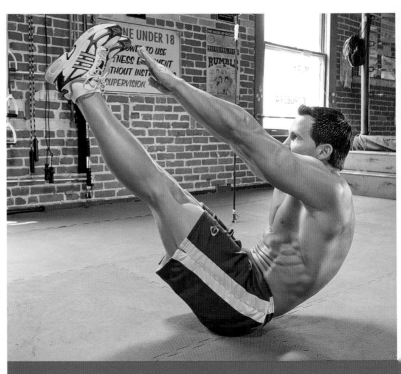

## TWISTING V-SIT
Lie faceup on the floor with your legs straight, arms at your sides, palms down. Raise your legs and torso 45 degrees off the floor to form a V. Reach your hands alongside your legs as high as you can without rounding your back. Hold, then twist slightly to the left to point your hands toward your left foot. Rotate back to center, then twist to the right. Alternate sides for reps.

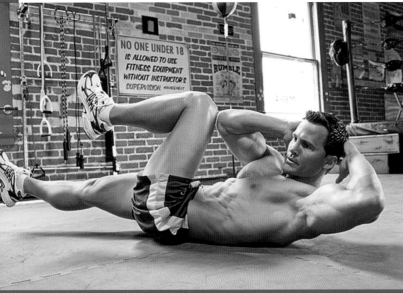

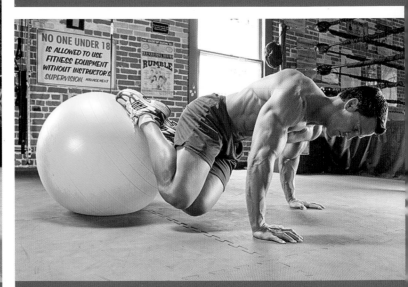

## BICYCLE
Lie faceup on the floor with your knees bent and feet together in the air. Place your fingers lightly behind your head. Draw your left knee toward your chest and extend your right leg. Simultaneously curl your torso up and twist to the left so your right elbow and left knee touch. Lower back to the floor, switch sides, and repeat.

## TWISTING EXERCISE-BALL KNEE TUCK
Get into pushup position with your shins up on an exercise ball. Keeping your legs together, slowly roll the ball forward by bending your knees. Draw your knees as close to your right elbow as you can, pause, then extend your legs back to the start. Alternate sides for reps.

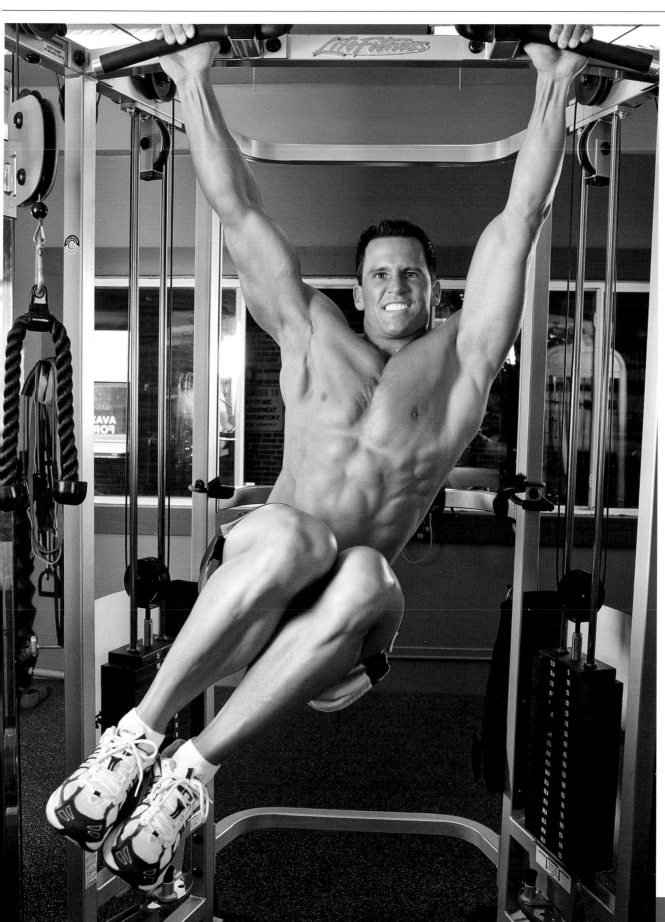

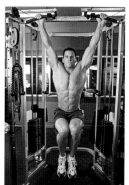

## HANGING KNEE TWIST

Hang freely from a pullup bar, hands wider than shoulder-width apart. Slowly raise your knees to the left as you tilt your pelvis upward. (Imagine you're trying to touch your right hip to your chest.) Pause, lower your legs, and repeat to the other side.

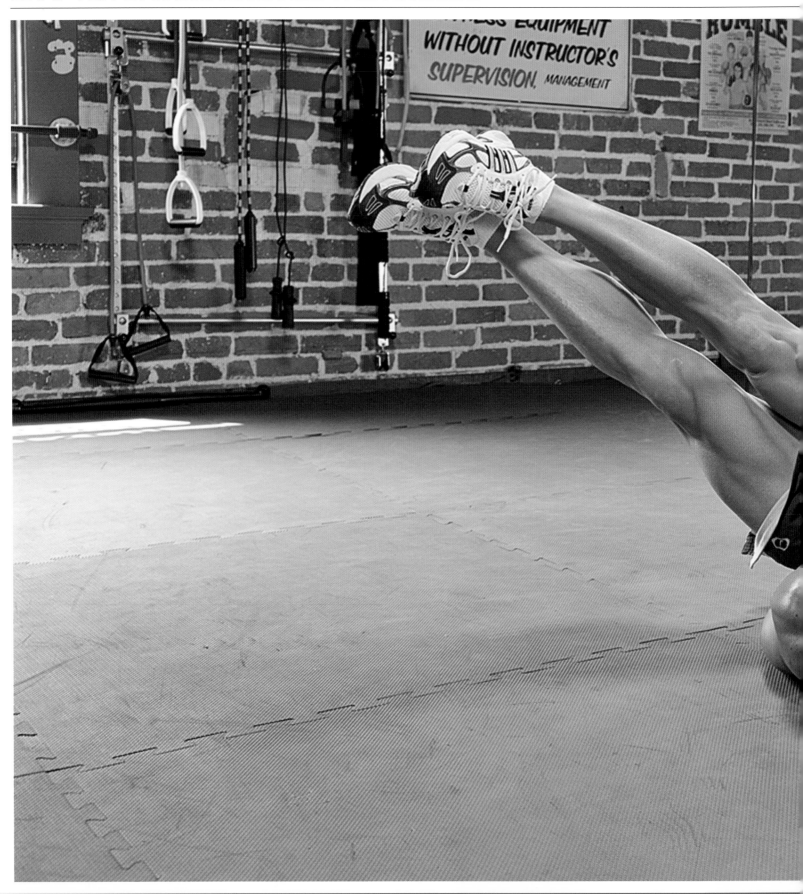

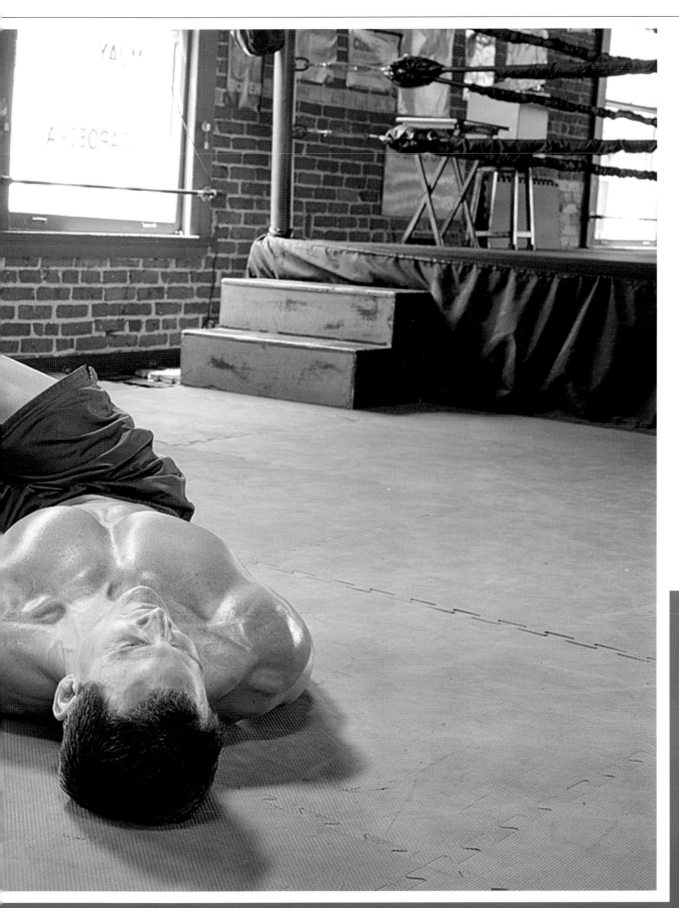

**WINDSHIELD WIPER**
Lie faceup on the floor, arms by your sides and hands tucked under your glutes, palms down. Draw your legs together and slowly raise them until your feet are perpendicular to the floor. Keeping your head and shoulders on the floor, slowly drop your legs to the left as far as you can, keeping them together. Pause, return to center, then drop your legs to the right. Alternate sides for reps.

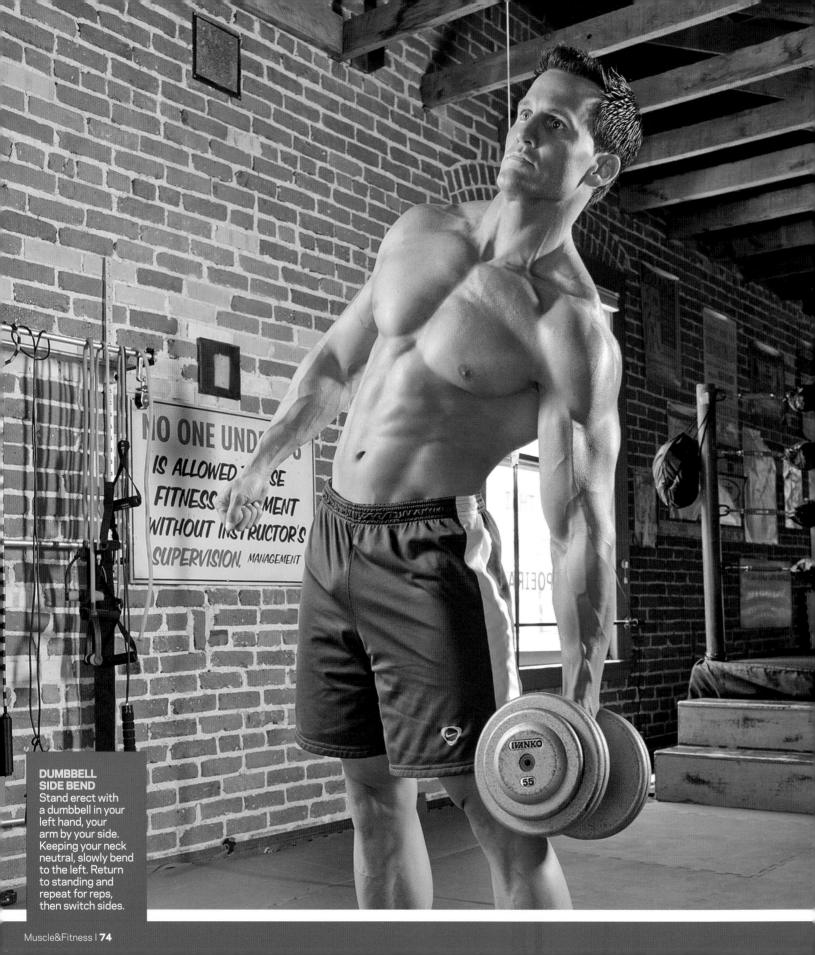

**DUMBBELL SIDE BEND**
Stand erect with a dumbbell in your left hand, your arm by your side. Keeping your neck neutral, slowly bend to the left. Return to standing and repeat for reps, then switch sides.

# BEND IT EXERCISES

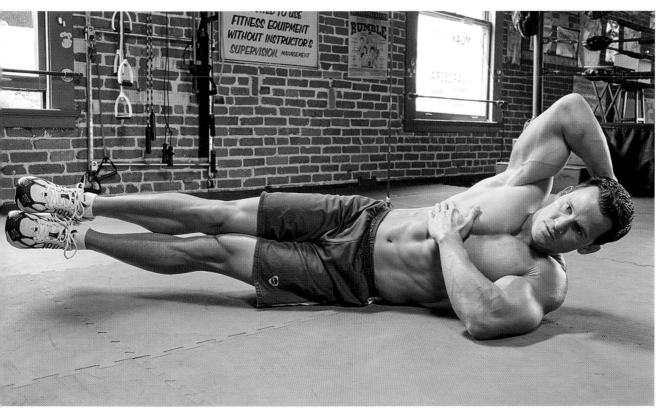

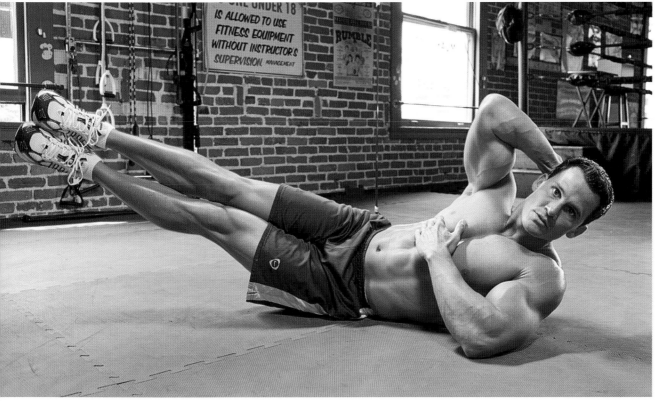

**DOUBLE JACKKNIFE**
Lie on your left side with your legs straight. Touch your right fingers lightly to the back of your head so your elbow points to the ceiling. Slowly raise both legs toward your right elbow. Pause, then lower back to the start. Repeat for reps, then switch sides.

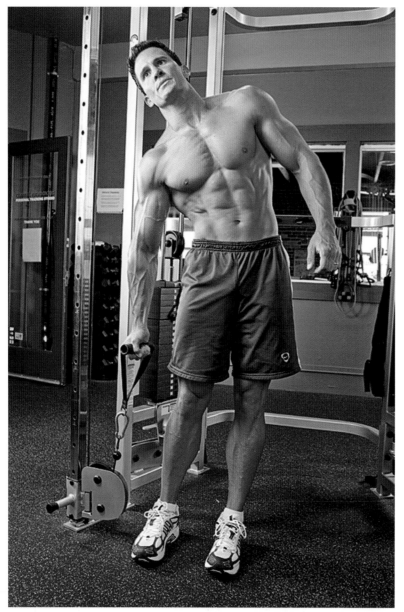

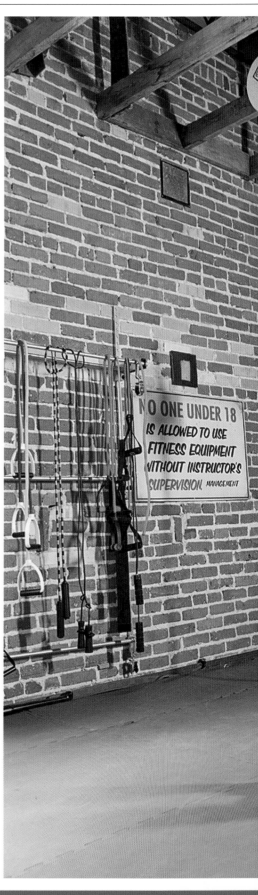

**CABLE SIDE BEND**
Attach a stirrup handle to a low-pulley cable and stand erect with your right side facing the weight stack. Grasp the handle in your right hand, keeping your arm by your side. With your head forward, slowly bend to the right. Return to standing and repeat for reps, then switch sides.

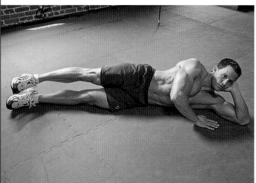

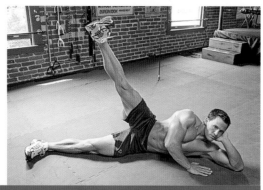

**ONE-LEG JACKKNIFE**
Lie on your left side and upper arm, and rest your head on your left hand. Place your right hand on the floor in front of you, bend your left knee slightly and raise your right leg an inch or two off the floor. Keeping your right leg straight, lift it as high as you can. Pause, then lower back to the start. Repeat for reps, then switch sides.

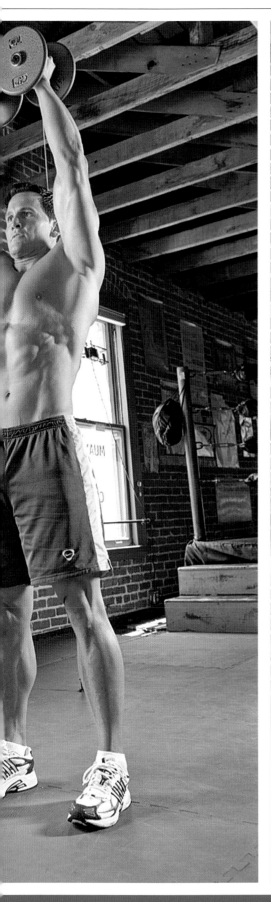

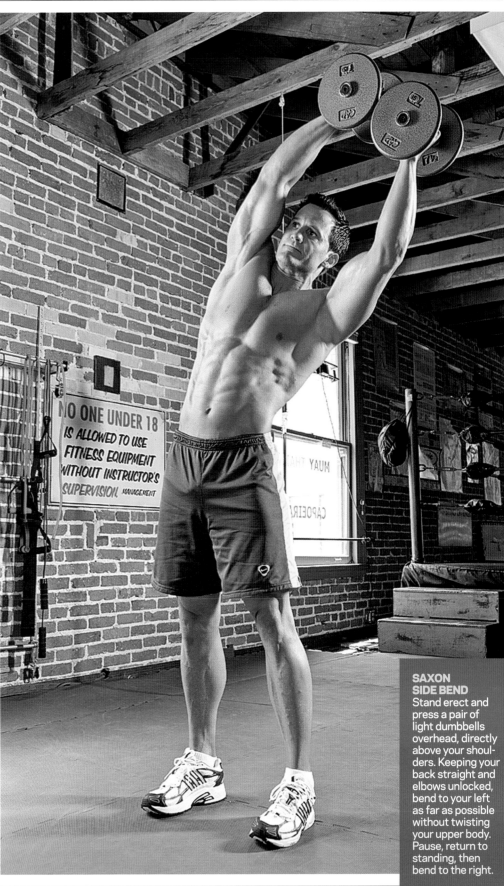

**SAXON SIDE BEND**
Stand erect and press a pair of light dumbbells overhead, directly above your shoulders. Keeping your back straight and elbows unlocked, bend to your left as far as possible without twisting your upper body. Pause, return to standing, then bend to the right.

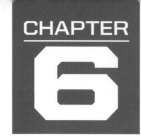

## CHAPTER 6

# OLD-SCHOOL ABS

**A former heavyweight contender shows you how to get a ripped midsection the old-fashioned way. This might sting a little.**

"**Y**ou're an evil son of a bitch."
It takes only a few minutes of speaking with heavyweight boxer turned trainer Justin Fortune to come to this realization. A faint smile crosses the affable Aussie's face, and you get the idea that this summation is one of the more benign epithets he has heard from a lifetime of days working in construction yards and nights spent first in powerlifting weight rooms and later in boxing gyms.

Without skipping a beat, he nods: "Absolutely."

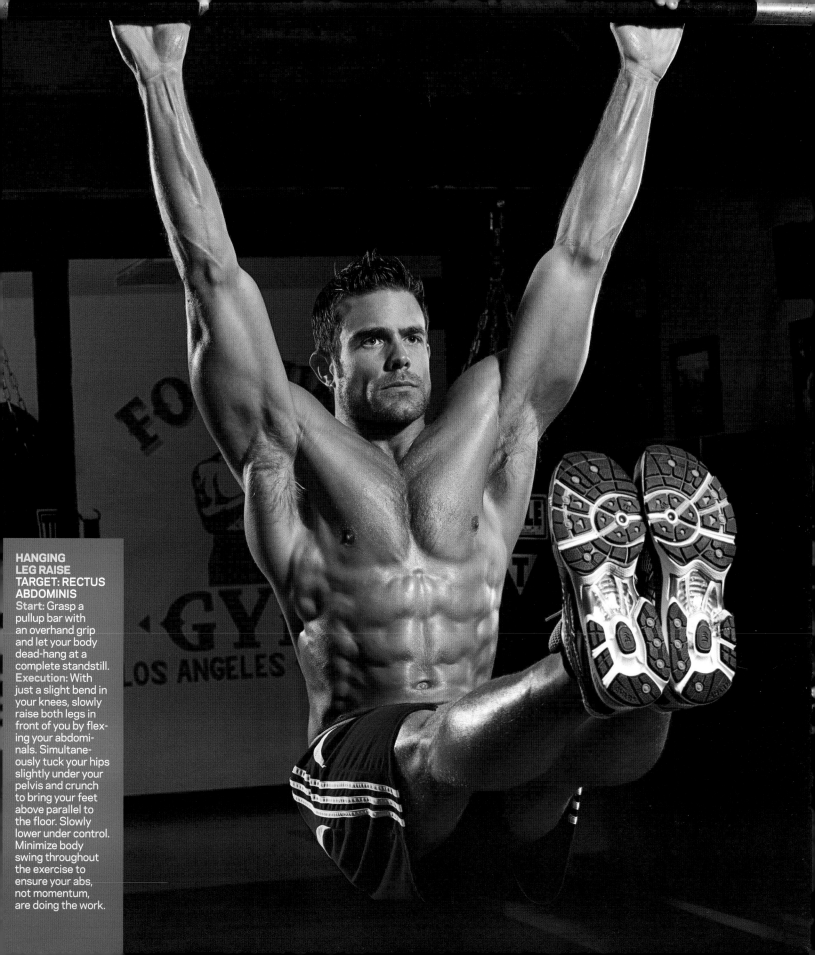

**HANGING LEG RAISE**
**TARGET: RECTUS ABDOMINIS**
Start: Grasp a pullup bar with an overhand grip and let your body dead-hang at a complete standstill. Execution: With just a slight bend in your knees, slowly raise both legs in front of you by flexing your abdominals. Simultaneously tuck your hips slightly under your pelvis and crunch to bring your feet above parallel to the floor. Slowly lower under control. Minimize body swing throughout the exercise to ensure your abs, not momentum, are doing the work.

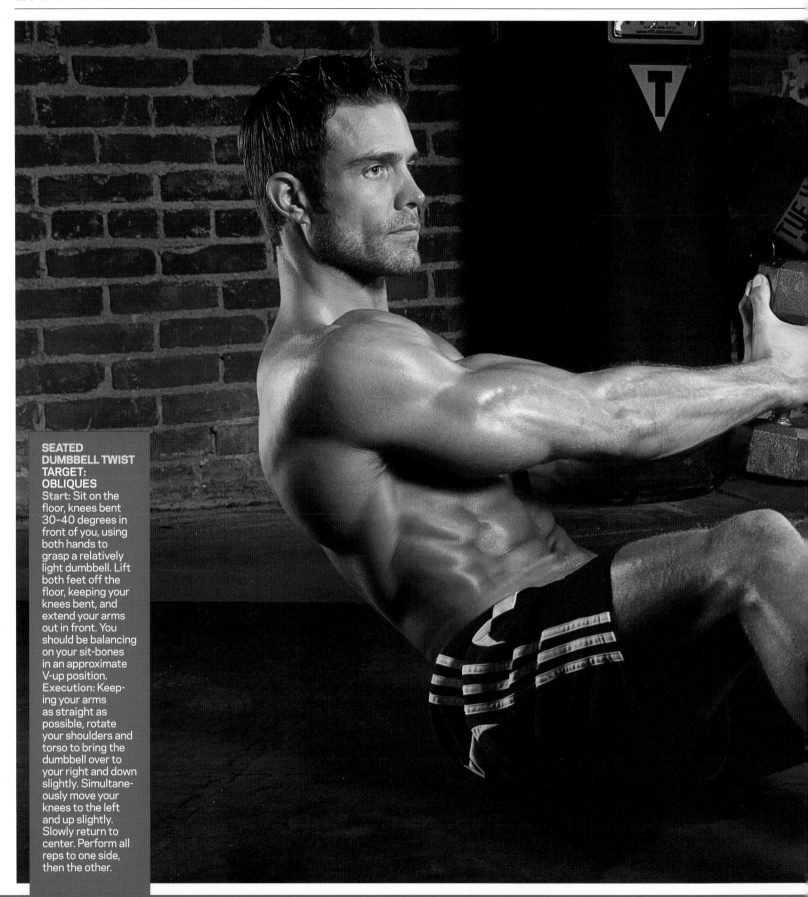

## SEATED DUMBBELL TWIST

**TARGET: OBLIQUES**

**Start:** Sit on the floor, knees bent 30–40 degrees in front of you, using both hands to grasp a relatively light dumbbell. Lift both feet off the floor, keeping your knees bent, and extend your arms out in front. You should be balancing on your sit-bones in an approximate V-up position.

**Execution:** Keeping your arms as straight as possible, rotate your shoulders and torso to bring the dumbbell over to your right and down slightly. Simultaneously move your knees to the left and up slightly. Slowly return to center. Perform all reps to one side, then the other.

# OLD SCHOOL MEETS NEW

Any loyal reader of *M&F* knows that changing up your workouts and shocking your muscles into growth is one of the cornerstones of developing your physique. The importance of overcoming plateaus can't be overstated. But when it comes to ab training, "shocking your system" is just another way of saying, "This is gonna hurt."

Fortune has become a master of devising training schemes that catch his clients unaware and painfully jolt them from whatever comfortable reverie they've lulled themselves into. Conjuring up painful cocktails of sets, reps, and unorthodox moves is more than a 9-to-5 job for Fortune; it's his passion. "I have a couple of Scotches and a cigar, and I watch fights and think of a bunch of horrible s—t that I can do to my people," he says. "That's exactly how I do it."

Fortune has a wealth of experience from which to draw. As a young man, he competed as a powerlifter before embarking on a professional boxing career that spanned 20 years and included a 1995 bout with then-heavyweight champion Lennox Lewis. He now owns and runs Fortune Gym in Hollywood, CA. His stable of clients includes actors, doctors, and lawyers, as well as seven pro boxers and four pro MMA fighters. His sinister ab creations are a combination of classic training techniques and some creative twists, with just a bit of basic manual labor thrown in for overall toughness and strength.

"Before I came to America, I was on the ass end of a 90-pound jackhammer, mixing mud or lifting bricks. I went to the gym at night, then I'd fight on the weekends, and I'd f—kin' smash people," Fortune says. "So my gym looks like a construction site. I use sandbags, water buckets, wheelbarrows full of stones, shovels. I have a tire with a big, old 6-inch shipping rope that [I have them] pull around."

While he routinely drops as many f-bombs in one conversation as he dropped opponents in the ring during his career, Fortune is no slurry punch-drunk palooka with a blind devotion to a long-gone era of fitness. For instance, he likes the hanging leg raise—an exercise boxers have been doing for hundreds of years—but he eschews moves that lack control, like the pugilistic tradition of dropping a medicine ball on an athlete's clenched abs and the lying leg raise in which a trainer throws the client's feet to the floor.

A feeling of tough love exudes from the gritty brick walls of Fortune Gym, and from its gritty owner. Even when he puts a weight plate on the back of a client holding a plank pose or hits another with a bamboo stick, his look of satisfaction belies more than mere sadism. "I got a lot of guys and girls who'll come in here and I'll bust them a new a-hole and they keep coming back," Fortune says. "I'll put a lot more time into them because they appreciate it. After about a month they see results, and that's the best part."

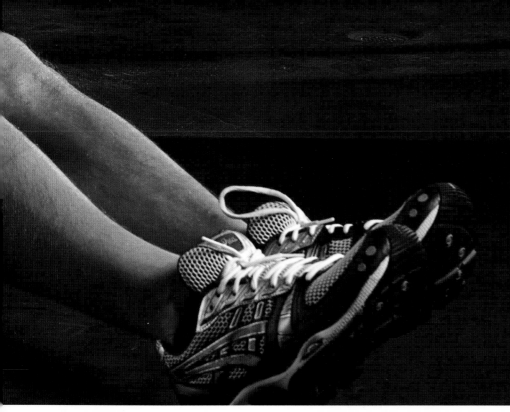

## THE ROUTINE

Conditioning expert Justin Fortune designed this program to hit all the usual abdominal muscle groups but with maximum unpredictability. It'll stress your core with weights, gravity and your body's own resistance. If you find it too difficult, just remember Fortune's encouraging words: "If you don't want to do it, then f—k off. Don't waste my time or yours."

| EXERCISE | SETS | REPS |
|---|---|---|
| Hanging Leg Raise | 4 | 15 |
| Seated Dumbbell Twist | 4 | 15 (per side) |
| Reverse Superman | 6 | To failure |
| Weighted Side Plank | 4 | 15 (per side) |
| Pike Plank | 3 | 10 |
| Stick Move* | 1 | Work up to 3 minutes |

*Optional

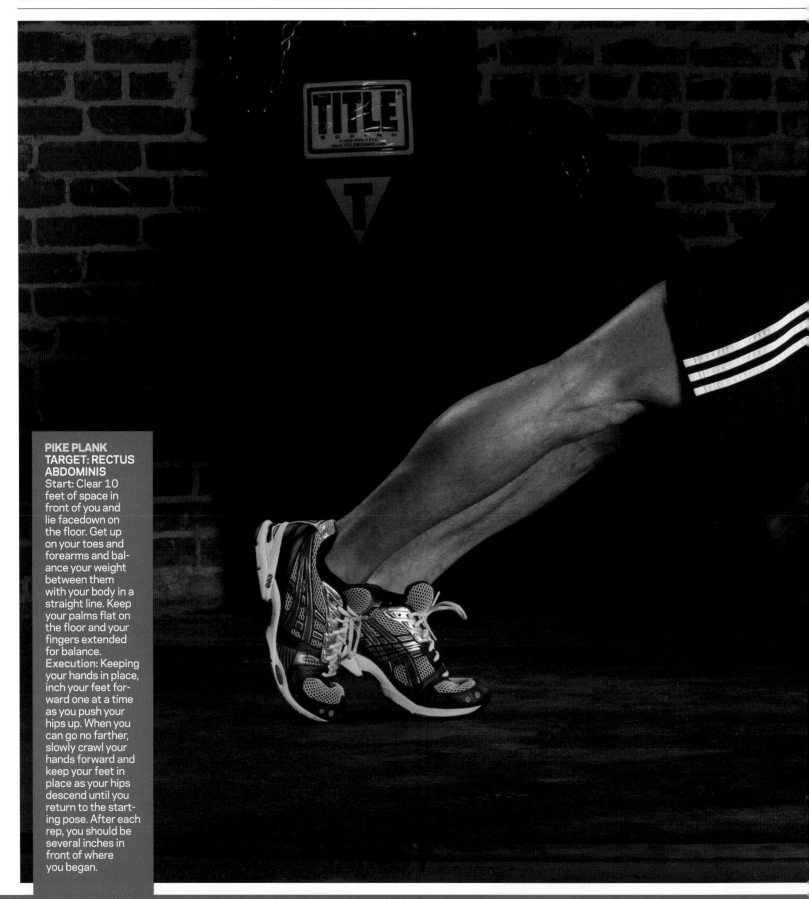

**PIKE PLANK**
**TARGET: RECTUS ABDOMINIS**

**Start:** Clear 10 feet of space in front of you and lie facedown on the floor. Get up on your toes and forearms and balance your weight between them with your body in a straight line. Keep your palms flat on the floor and your fingers extended for balance.

**Execution:** Keeping your hands in place, inch your feet forward one at a time as you push your hips up. When you can go no farther, slowly crawl your hands forward and keep your feet in place as your hips descend until you return to the starting pose. After each rep, you should be several inches in front of where you began.

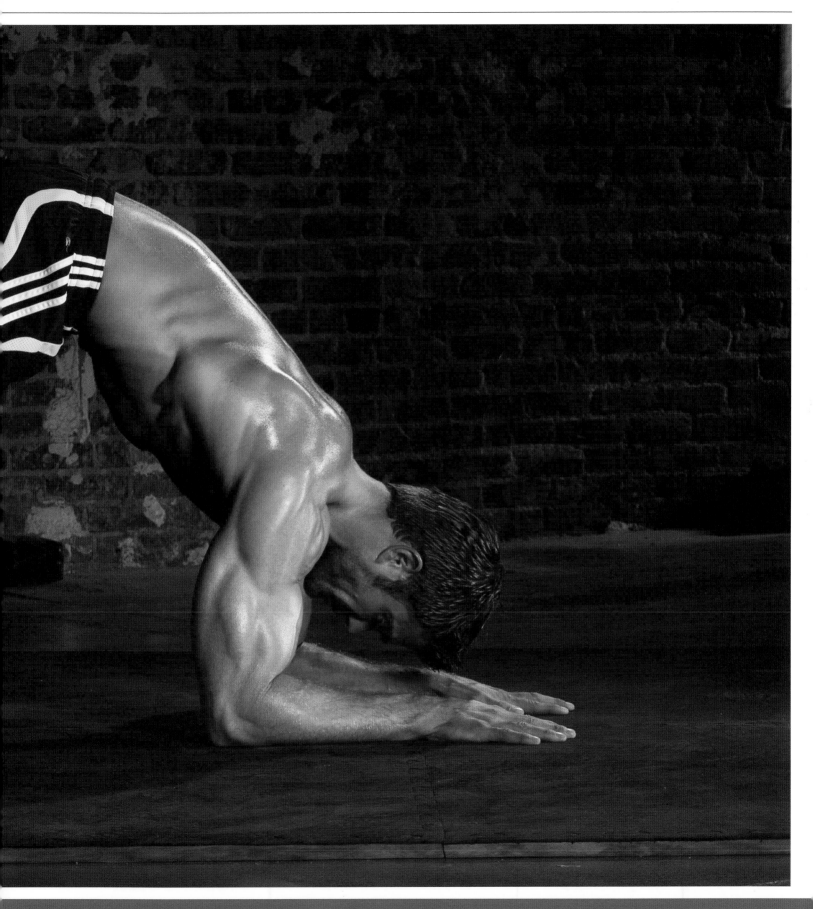

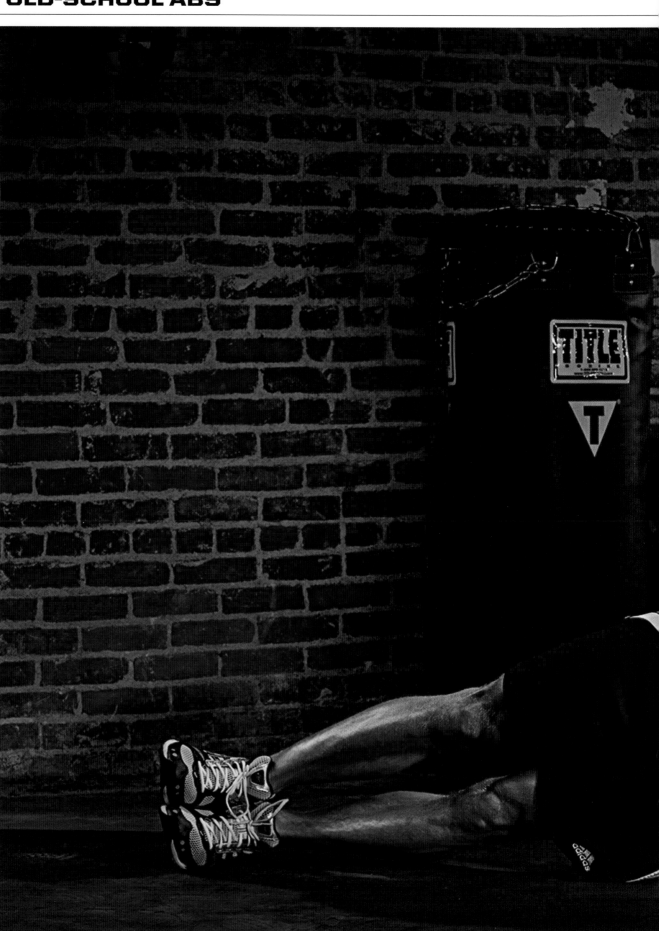

**WEIGHTED SIDE PLANK**
**TARGET:**
**OBLIQUES**
**Start:** Grasp a 5-pound weight in your right hand and lie on the floor on your left elbow and forearm, stacking your feet so your body creates a straight line. Raise your hips off the floor so you're supporting yourself on your forearm and left foot, creating a straight line from head to toe. Extend your right arm toward the ceiling. Keep your head aligned with your spine at all times. **Execution:** Keeping your right arm straight, slowly bring the weight down in an arc, rotating your torso so your abs turn toward the floor at the bottom of the move. The toes of your top foot will touch the floor for balance. When your right arm comes to parallel to the floor, hold the pose for a beat before slowly returning to the start position.

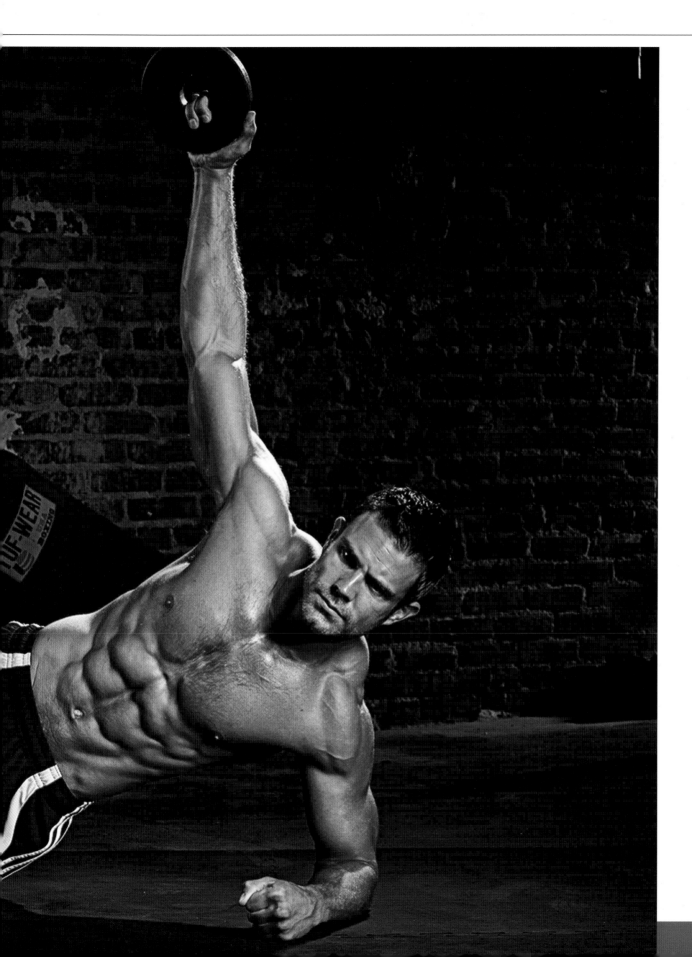

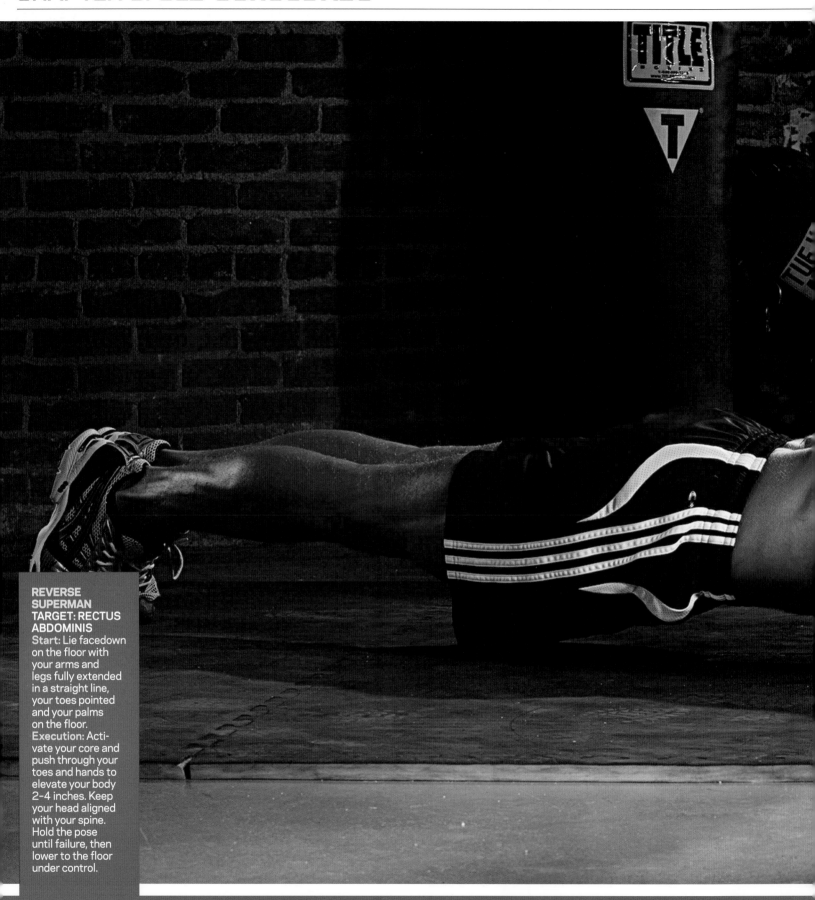

**REVERSE SUPERMAN**
**TARGET: RECTUS ABDOMINIS**
Start: Lie facedown on the floor with your arms and legs fully extended in a straight line, your toes pointed and your palms on the floor.
Execution: Activate your core and push through your toes and hands to elevate your body 2–4 inches. Keep your head aligned with your spine. Hold the pose until failure, then lower to the floor under control.

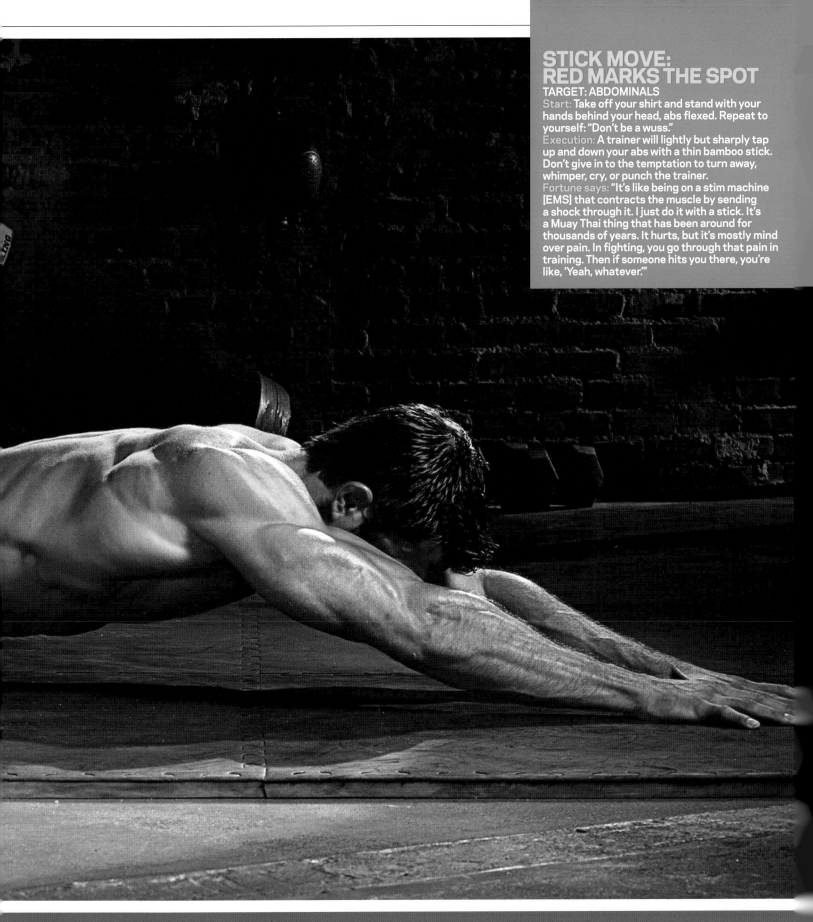

## STICK MOVE: RED MARKS THE SPOT
### TARGET: ABDOMINALS

**Start:** Take off your shirt and stand with your hands behind your head, abs flexed. Repeat to yourself: "Don't be a wuss."

**Execution:** A trainer will lightly but sharply tap up and down your abs with a thin bamboo stick. Don't give in to the temptation to turn away, whimper, cry, or punch the trainer.

**Fortune says:** "It's like being on a stim machine [EMS] that contracts the muscle by sending a shock through it. I just do it with a stick. It's a Muay Thai thing that has been around for thousands of years. It hurts, but it's mostly mind over pain. In fighting, you go through that pain in training. Then if someone hits you there, you're like, 'Yeah, whatever.'"

# CHAPTER 7

# GUT

**Keep your abs guessing—and your six-pack progressing— with this intuitive midsection routine.**

When it comes to ab training, Gunnar Peterson, C.S.C.S., isn't all that impressed by big numbers. Those who do marathon sets of crunches and leg raises may build some muscular endurance, but their quest for a chiseled washboard is futile.

"I think the most common flaw in abdominal programs is the high number of crunches people perform," says Peterson, whose Beverly Hills facility is a training haven for elite athletes and Hollywood celebrities alike. "I'm a fan of the crunch, but the abs must be trained in all three planes of motion, with weight, and from a number of different positions. You have to mix it up constantly."

If anyone knows how to mix things up, it's Peterson. This is obvious the minute you step into his gym and see at least a dozen machines you never even knew existed. All this novel equipment is especially helpful when training abs.

"Think about the muscles in the abdominal wall and in the core in general— they get worked all the time," he states. "They're the first muscles to fire with any movement, and they constantly stabilize to keep you upright. So considering what these muscles go through on a daily basis, it requires a lot to really shock them. I don't think doing 250, 500, or even 1,000 crunches is enough when you look at how complex the musculature is; it's like giving a spelling-bee champion a bunch of monosyllabic words. You've got to challenge those muscles. You have to throw them curveballs to make them react. And that's what I try to do here at the gym."

While Peterson's all about variety when it comes to working abs, he also believes in training instinctively. He's loathe to prescribe a finite number of sets and reps for a given workout. Instead, his broad guidelines for training the midsection are 6–20 total sets, varying the resistance so you do 6–25 reps per set.

"I'm not trying to give you a Fenway-size ballpark answer [for sets and reps], but it's different for every individual," he explains. "It depends on where you are in your program: Is it just a core day? Is it the third time you've hit abs that week? You want to push yourself, but some days you can't push too hard, and other days you can push all the way through because maybe you have three days of rest coming up. If you've been [training] for any amount of time, you should be able to feel your way through it.

"And when I say do 6–20 total sets of anywhere from 6–25 reps, that doesn't mean do 20 sets of 25 reps," he adds. "But it doesn't mean do six sets of six, either. You have to learn to be intuitive."

As you'll see on the following pages, Peterson's exercise suggestions utilize some unique and tough-to-find equipment. If your gym has some of it, great; if not, try the gym-friendly version listed for each one. The overall theme of the routine is to hit the abs from every conceivable angle with different machines and body weight exercises, varying loads, dropsets, you name it. "The more you mix things up," says Peterson, "the more your abs will respond to your training and the more attainable that elusive six-pack will be."

# INSTINCT

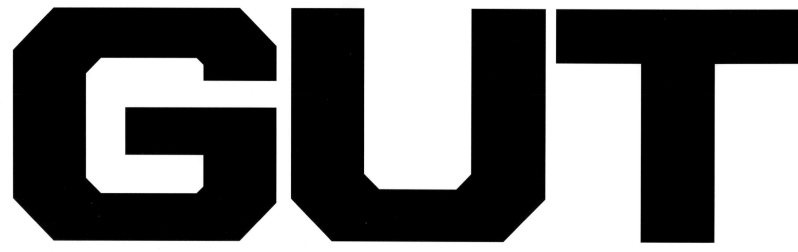

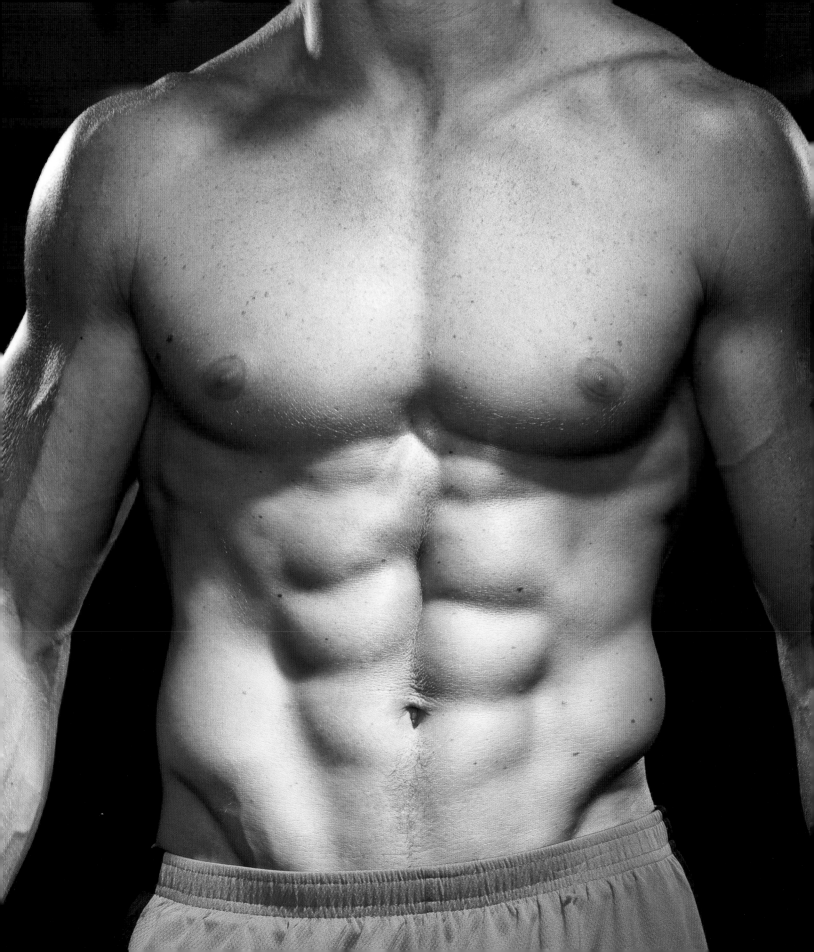

## THE WORKOUT

>> Of the following exercises, choose two to three per workout for anywhere from 6–20 total sets, depending on your experience level and being mindful not to overtrain.

>> Vary the resistance so you do 6–25 reps per set. On one exercise, for example, you might do three sets of 20, while on another you may do 4–5 sets of 6–10. Continually mix things up.

>> Train abs two to four days per week, adjusting your training volume accordingly: The more days per week you train abs, the lower the total sets should be per workout.

## EXERCISE MENU

VersaPulley Crunch (while kneeling on a BOSU)

Hanging Reverse Crunch
(with a corkscrew at the top)

Rotating Roman-Chair Crunch (with a Body Bar)

*Rocky IV* Reverse Crunch
(on a Louie Simmons Reverse Hyper)

Strive Machine Crunch (with cam-shift dropsets)

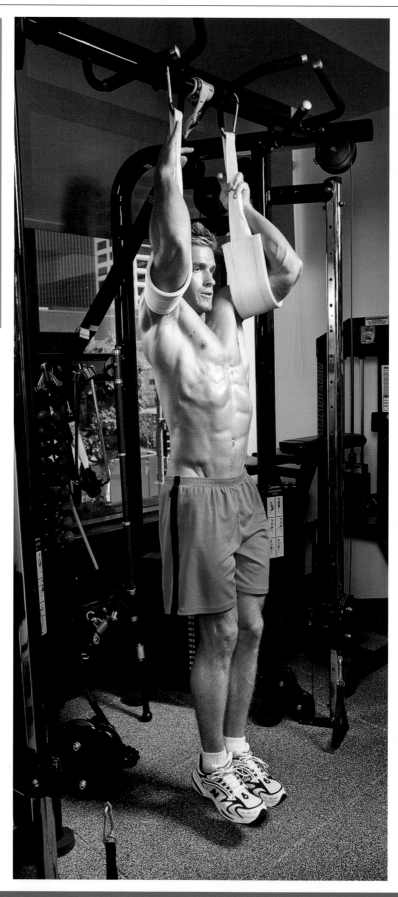

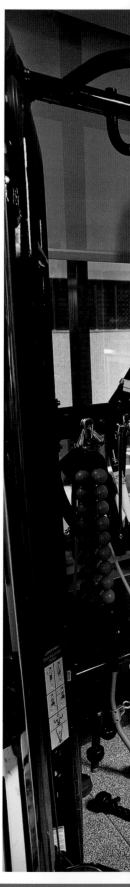

## HANGING REVERSE CRUNCH (WITH A CORKSCREW AT THE TOP)
### TARGETS: LOWER ABS, OBLIQUES

**Start:** Attach ab straps to a pullup bar or the top of a power rack. Place your triceps and elbows on the padded surface to support your weight. Grasp the top of the straps (close to the metal clips) and let your legs hang straight toward the floor.

**Execution:** In a powerful motion, bend your knees 90 degrees while simultaneously contracting your abs to lift your knees toward your elbows. As you reach the top, twist your torso ("corkscrew") so your knees point to one side. Drop your legs to the start position and repeat for reps, alternating sides.

**Gunnar's take:** "I push for a full range of motion on these. If it's too much, just go as high as you can and work your way up as you get stronger. The corkscrew motion calls into play the serratus muscles and obliques."

**Gym-friendly version:** This exercise can be performed at any gym with ab straps and a pullup bar high enough to allow for a full range of motion—make sure you can fully extend your legs at the bottom.

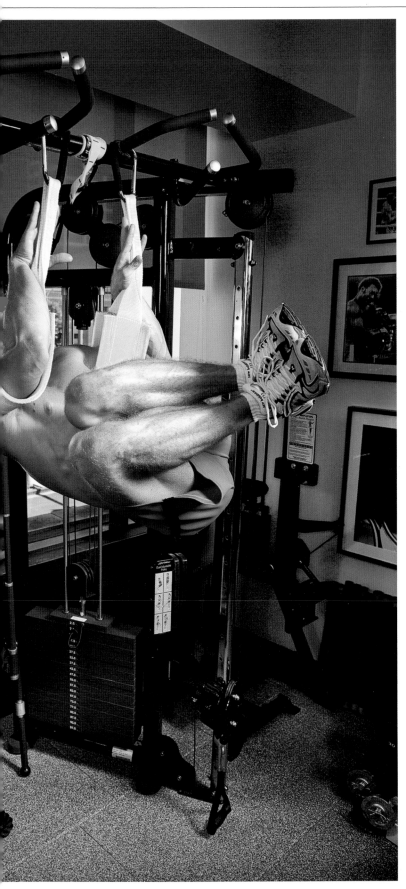
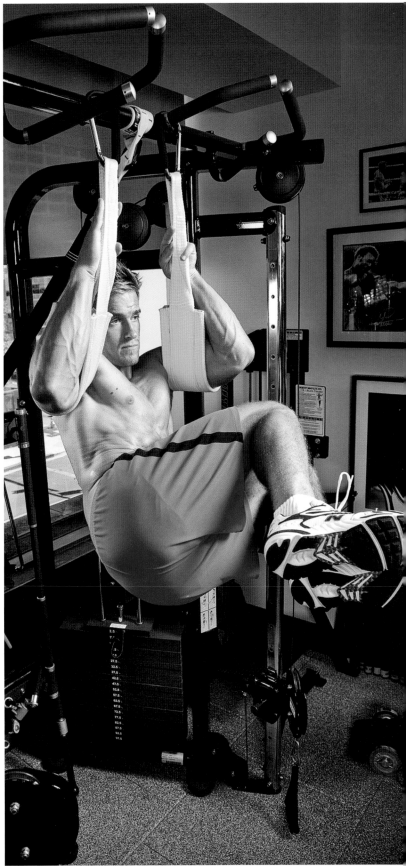

## VERSAPULLEY CRUNCH (WHILE KNEELING ON A BOSU)
### TARGET: UPPER ABS

**Start:** Kneel on the dome of a BOSU placed a couple of feet in front of a VersaPulley machine. Grasp the rope or handles with your upper arms alongside your head, and begin with your knees at 90-degree angles and your torso at roughly a 45-degree angle to the floor.

**Execution:** In an explosive motion, crunch your abs to bring your elbows to the BOSU, keeping your arms in position and your hands close to your head. Resist the negative by keeping your abs tight and not letting the machine pull you back up too fast.

**Gunnar's take:** "I love the eccentric on the VersaPulley. Whatever you take from the machine on the concentric portion, it gives right back on the eccentric. If more relationships had that kind of give and take, the divorce rate would be cut in half. Using the BOSU increases the range of motion at the bottom because your knees are elevated, and it challenges your stability and works the core more."

**Gym-friendly version:** A cable crunch mimics this movement but doesn't provide the same eccentric action you get with the VersaPulley. A better alternative is to secure a thick rubber band to the top of a power rack or other stable structure, grasp the bottom of the band and perform the same movement. Because of the band's elasticity, it'll pull you up faster than a cable, forcing you to resist the negative that much more.

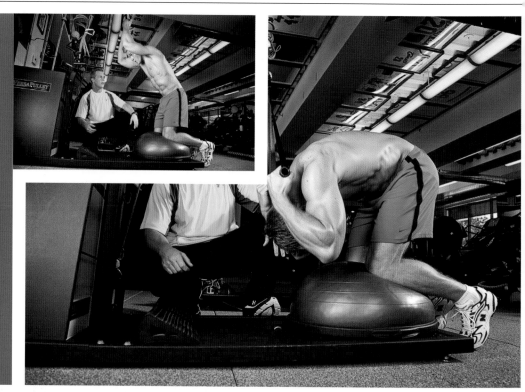

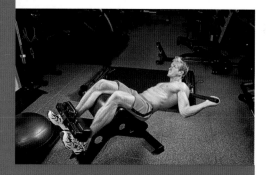

## ROTATING ROMAN-CHAIR CRUNCH (WITH A BODY BAR)
### TARGETS: UPPER ABS, OBLIQUES

**Start:** Sit more or less erect on a roman chair with your feet secured. Hold a Body Bar (or any lightweight bar) across your upper traps with your hands wide.

**Execution:** At a relatively quick pace—one second up, one second down—do full situps. Go down as far as you can and return all the way to the start while twisting to one side; alternate sides for reps.

**Gunnar's take:** "This stresses your abs while moving in two planes. When you sit up and twist, that's a move you do all the time; in fact, you do it every morning when you get out of bed. Athletes in a number of sports do it, so it's great to train like that."

**Gym-friendly version:** If your gym doesn't have a roman chair, use a decline bench at the steepest setting. If this limits how far you can descend, especially since the bar will get in the way, hold either a light dumbbell or medicine ball at chest level or overhead. "Adding the extra load makes you really feel it," Peterson says. "It'll be much more challenging."

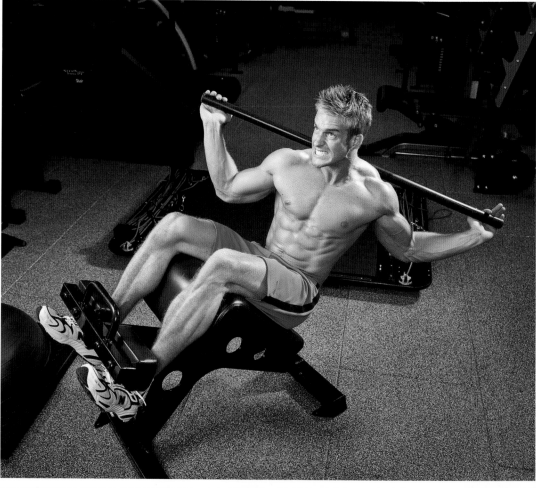

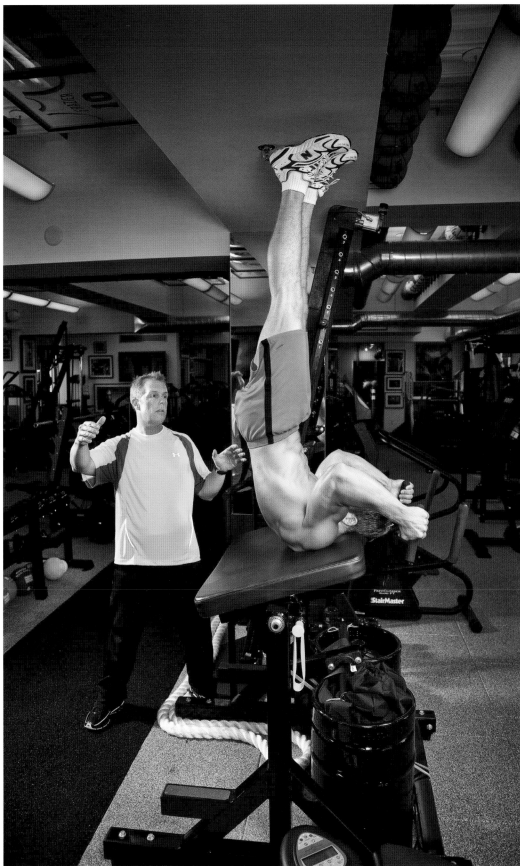

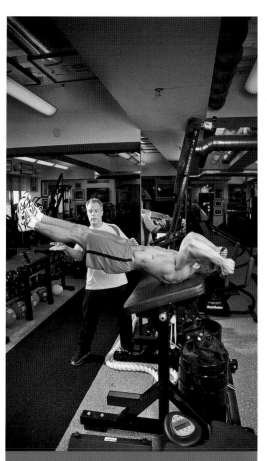

## ROCKY IV REVERSE CRUNCH
### (ON A LOUIE SIMMONS REVERSE HYPER)
### TARGETS: LOWER ABS, CORE

**Start:** Lie faceup on the bench with your back flat on the pad. Grasp the handles overhead and begin with your legs extended in line with your torso.

**Execution:** Contract your abs to raise your feet toward the ceiling. Your lower back should come off the bench as you crunch your abs to bring your pelvis closer to your ribcage. Lower yourself slowly, resisting the negative as much as possible.

**Gunnar's take:** "This is basically a leg raise, but you focus on the negative by lowering slowly. And you can go all the way up on your scapula, just like Rocky did when he was training in Russia in *Rocky IV*."

**Gym-friendly version:** Not many gyms have a Louie Simmons reverse hyper bench. The logical substitute is a standard decline bench, though it won't allow for quite as much range of motion at the bottom of the move.

CHAPTER 7: GUT INSTINCT

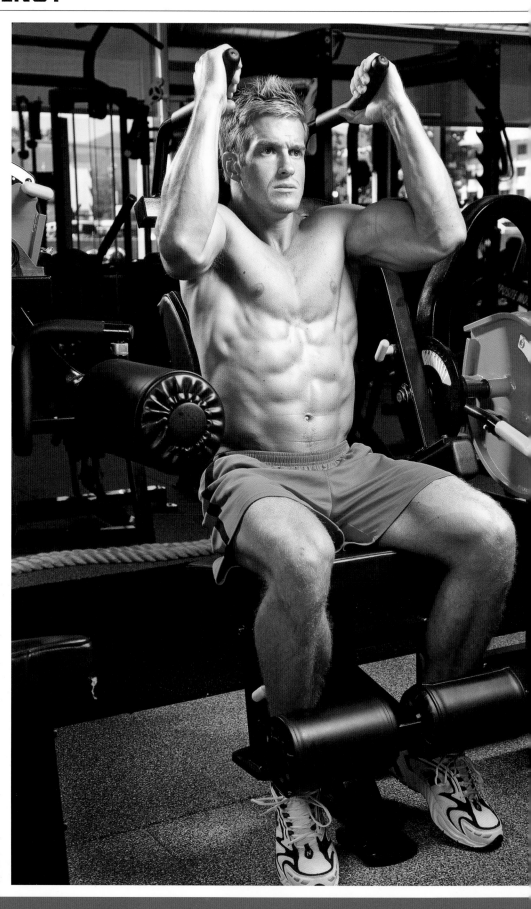

**STRIVE MACHINE CRUNCH
(WITH CAM-SHIFT DROPSETS)
TARGET: UPPER ABS**

**Start:** Place the machine's cam setting at the Set 3 position—this provides more resistance at the beginning of the range of motion (ROM)—and choose a moderately heavy resistance on the weight stack. Sit erect with your back flat and grasp the handles overhead.

**Execution:** Rep out to failure by crunching your ribcage toward your pelvis. Immediately change the cam setting to the Set 1 position—this provides more resistance at the middle of the ROM—and rep to failure again. Immediately change the cam setting to the Set 2 position—which provides more resistance at the end of the ROM—and rep to failure. That's one set.

**Gunnar's take:** "Sometimes when doing dropsets on a regular cam machine you'll find that you still have something left, but not where the machine stresses you in the range of motion. The Strive machine allows you to drop the cam setting without changing the weight, so you can eke out more reps without having to go lighter. This helps you get more out of every set."

**Gym-friendly version:** The cam machines in most health clubs don't feature adjustable varying resistance like Strive machines do. The best way to mimic this is on an old-school slantboard or adjustable decline bench. Peterson suggests starting at the steepest decline and doing 10 reps, then dropping to a medium decline for 15 reps, then to the smallest decline for 20 reps.

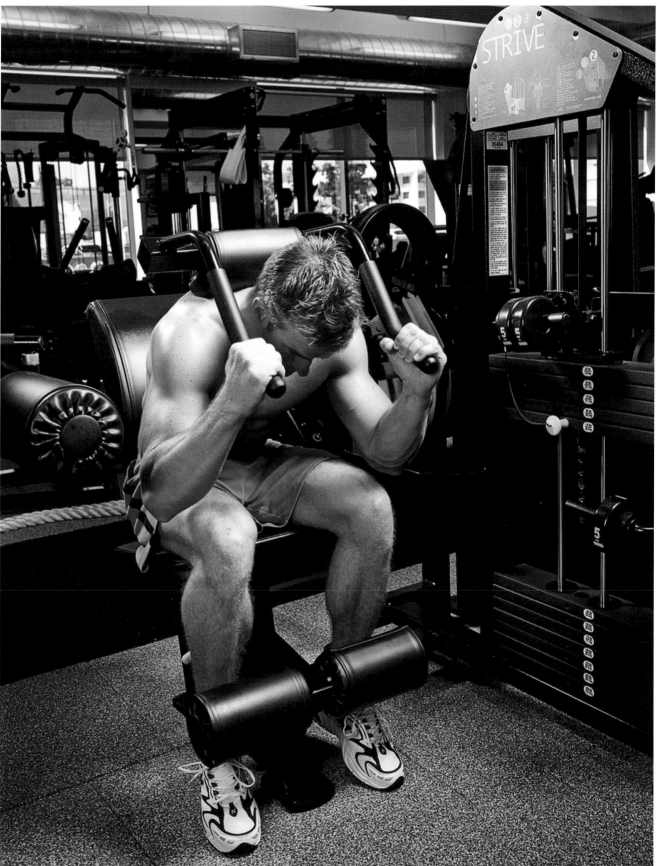
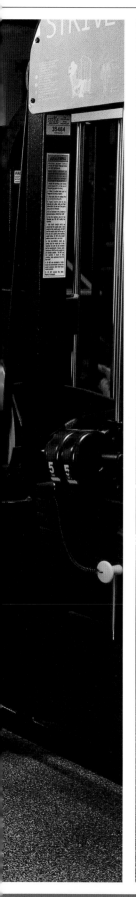

# THE NO-CRUNCH CORE WORKOUT

**Walk away from overused ab moves and develop a real core of steel with this unorthodox training plan.**

C onsider this: Your core may not be strong enough to support your training program.

Your middle sets the stage for your muscular limbs to perform. From overhead squats to upright rows, a weak core will fold like a house of cards even if your arms and legs are more than strong enough to lift a weight.

"Think of shooting a cannonball off a canoe. It's just going to blow up the canoe, and the ball will go two feet," says Zac Woodfin, C.S.C.S., performance specialist at Athletes' Performance in Los Angeles. "If you shoot it off a solid-steel battleship, on the other hand, you can launch the same cannonball hundreds of feet, if not farther."

To make consistent and steady gains in the gym, and to protect yourself from injury, you need a core of steel. But what makes up this crucial region? It's more complicated than you might think. For the purposes of this workout, we'll focus on the abdominals and the muscles that support the pelvis and the thoraco-lumbar spine—essentially your spine from your pelvis to (but not including) shoulders.

"A primary role of the core is supporting the spine," explains William Whiting, Ph.D., C.S.C.S., professor of kinesiology at California State University-Northridge. "One important element is to emphasize different types of core training, with perhaps endurance being initially preferred over strength. Because in certain tasks involving limb movements, it's vital that the core act as a rigid body to allow a stable foundation."

In other words, while the body performs a certain task, the core must maintain an isometric contraction to stabilize the spine and not move. This favors endurance, and these eight exercises were chosen to help build the stable, enduring core that you need to enhance the rest of your training.

To get the most from this program, add one exercise per body part to your current workout to make sure your core doesn't get the day off. You can perform the move at the beginning or end of your routine, when the target muscle is already fatigued. Keep in mind that you want to train your core to stabilize your spine, so use a moderately heavy weight that allows you to complete 10–12 reps. Just don't lift more weight than your core can handle—you don't want your battleship to resemble a canoe.

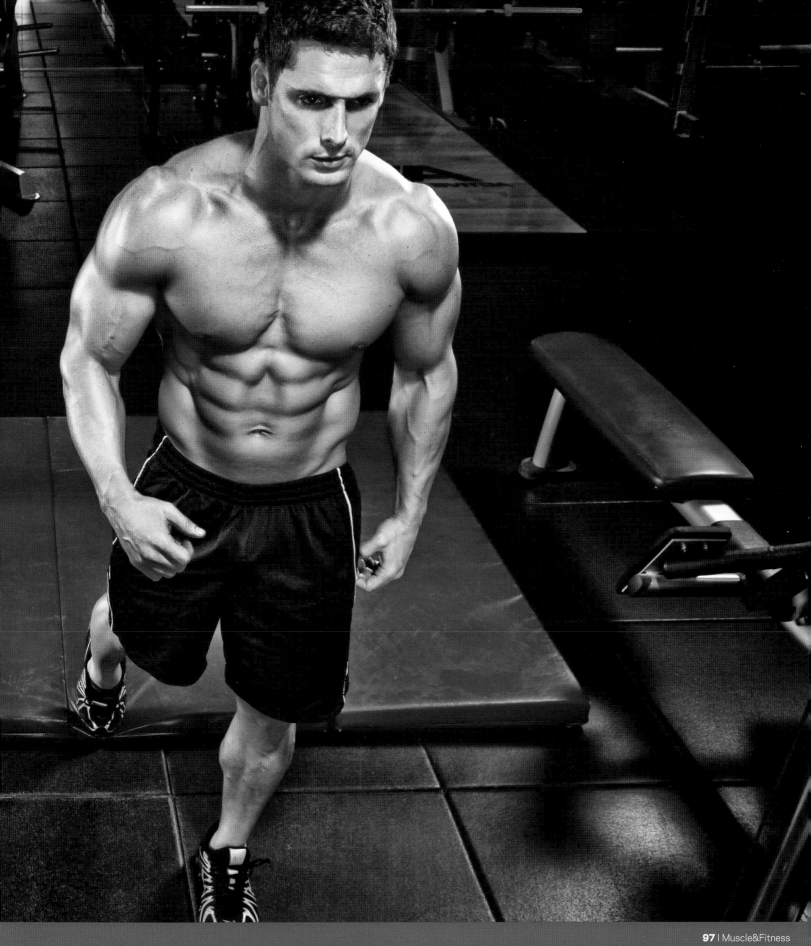

## THE PROGRAM

**Add one exercise per body part to your current workout at either the beginning or end of your routine. Use a moderately heavy weight.**

| EXERCISE | SETS | REPS |
|---|---|---|
| **CHEST** | | |
| One-Arm Cable Press | 3 | 10–12 per side |
| Alternating Dumbbell Press (with hips off bench) | 3 | 10–12 per side |
| **BACK** | | |
| One-Leg, One-Arm Bentover Dumbbell Row | 3 | 10–12 per side |
| Pullup (with hips and knees flexed 90 degrees) | 3 | To failure |
| **LEGS** | | |
| One-Leg Squat | 3 | 10–12 per side |
| One-Leg Romanian Deadlift | 3 | 10–12 per side |
| **SHOULDERS** | | |
| One-Leg Alternating Arnold Press | 3 | 10–12 per side |
| **FULL BODY** | | |
| Turkish Get-Up | 3 | 3–5 per side |

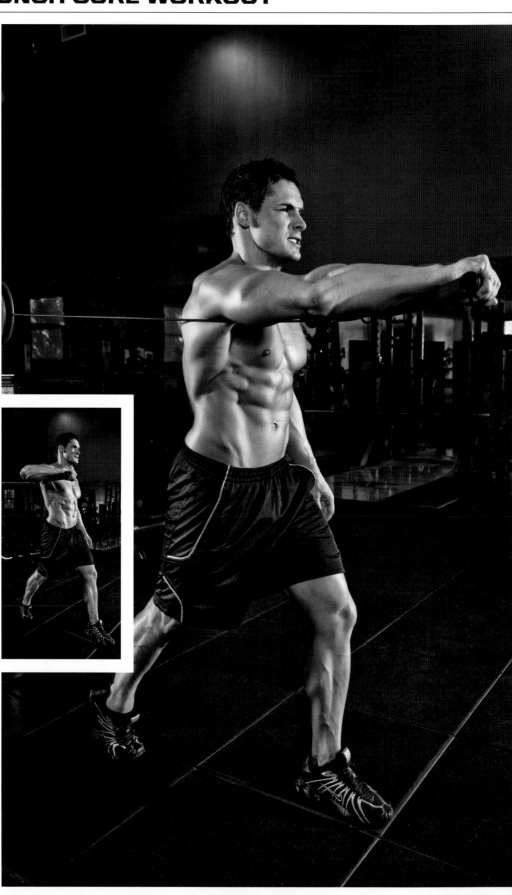

# CHEST

## ONE-ARM CABLE PRESS

>> **Start:** Attach a D-handle to the cable and adjust the pulley to slightly below shoulder level. Grasp the handle and face away from the weight stack so the cable runs under your arm. Stagger your stance with your nonworking-side foot in front and your feet in line. Most of your body weight should be on your front foot. Keep your torso erect, your core tight, and your spine neutral.

>> **Execution:** Using an overhand grip with the handle at upper-pec level, bring your elbow out to your side with your upper arm at a roughly 45-degree angle to your torso. Press forward to full-arm extension, preventing movement at your hips and core as much as possible. Repeat for reps, then switch sides. To increase the difficulty, bring your feet closer together.

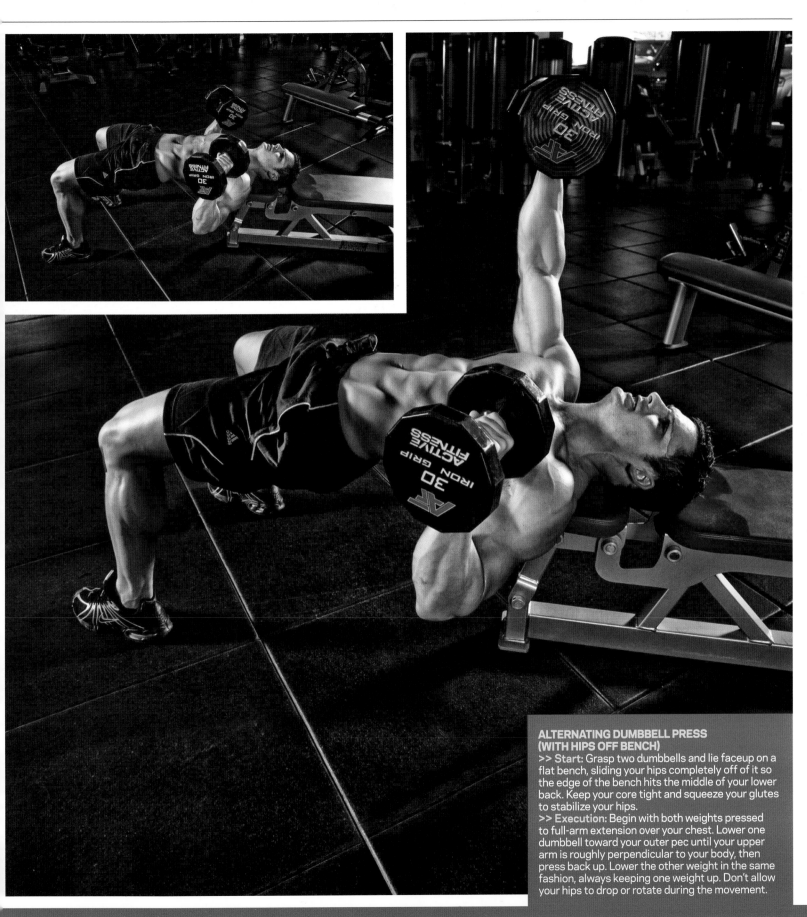

## ALTERNATING DUMBBELL PRESS (WITH HIPS OFF BENCH)

>> **Start:** Grasp two dumbbells and lie faceup on a flat bench, sliding your hips completely off of it so the edge of the bench hits the middle of your lower back. Keep your core tight and squeeze your glutes to stabilize your hips.

>> **Execution:** Begin with both weights pressed to full-arm extension over your chest. Lower one dumbbell toward your outer pec until your upper arm is roughly perpendicular to your body, then press back up. Lower the other weight in the same fashion, always keeping one weight up. Don't allow your hips to drop or rotate during the movement.

# BACK

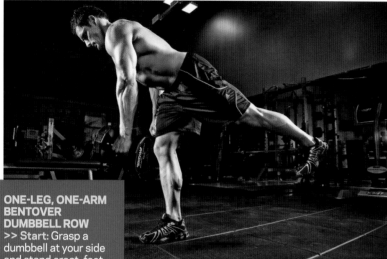
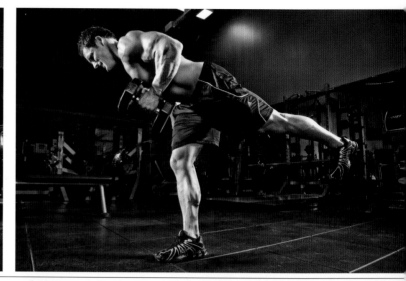

## ONE-LEG, ONE-ARM BENTOVER DUMBBELL ROW

>> Start: Grasp a dumbbell at your side and stand erect, feet together. Lift your working-side foot a couple of inches and pull your toes toward your shin. Keep your other knee slightly bent and grip the floor with your big toe for balance. Lean forward at the hips until your torso is between 45 degrees and parallel to the floor; your working leg should swing back so your body forms a straight line from head to ankle. Extend your working arm toward the floor.

>> Execution: Maintaining this bent-over position, pull the weight toward your hip in a rowing motion. Return to full-arm extension, repeat for reps, then switch arms and legs.

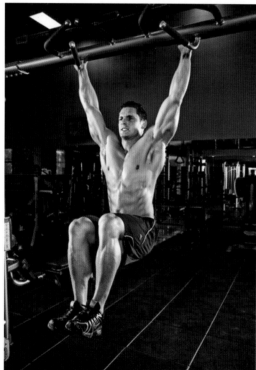
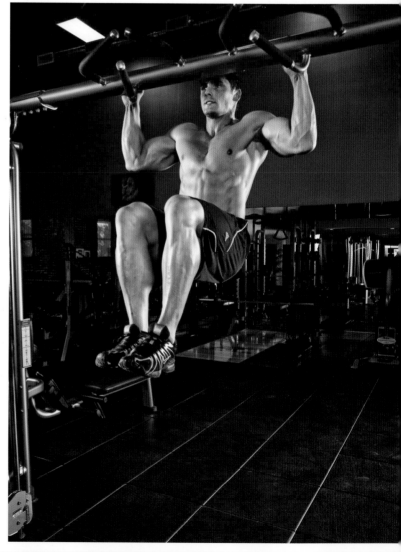

## PULLUP (WITH HIPS AND KNEES FLEXED 90 DEGREES)

>> Start: Grasp a pullup bar with an overhand grip, hands wider than shoulder width. Bend at the hips so your thighs are parallel to the floor and bend your knees 90 degrees. Point your toes up. Keep your core tight and your spine neutral.

>> Execution: Keeping your torso erect, contract your lats and squeeze your shoulder blades together to lift your chest to the bar. Slowly return to the start while maintaining your hip and leg position.

# LEGS

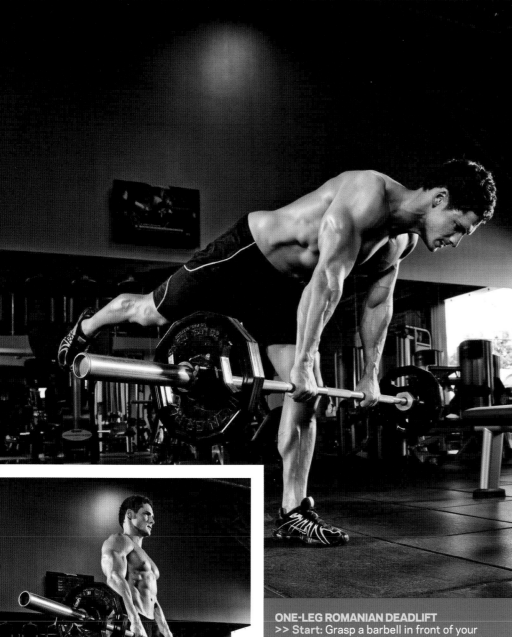

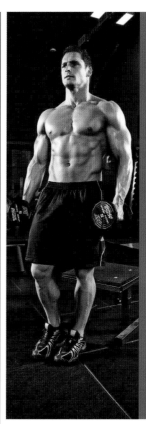

## ONE-LEG SQUAT
>> **Start:** Grasp two very light dumbbells at your sides as a counterbalance, and stand erect with your feet hip-width apart facing away from a flat bench. Keeping your core tight, lift one foot a couple of inches off the floor.
>> **Execution:** Bend your knees and hips to descend into a squat while simultaneously raising the weights in front of you to shoulder level. Control your working leg so your knee doesn't drift inward. At the bottom you should be level with or a couple of inches above the bench with your arms extended. Return to standing as you lower your arms to your sides. Repeat for reps, then switch sides.

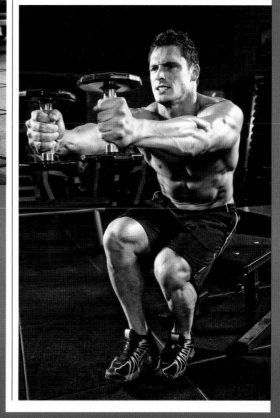

## ONE-LEG ROMANIAN DEADLIFT
>> **Start:** Grasp a barbell in front of your thighs and stand erect, feet together. Make your body as tall as possible. Lift one foot a couple of inches off the floor and pull your toes toward your shin. Keep your other knee slightly bent and grip the floor with your big toe for balance.
>> **Execution:** Lean forward at the hips until your torso is between 45 degrees and parallel to the floor; your nonworking leg should swing back so your body forms a straight line from head to ankle. Simultaneously extend your arms toward the floor, and keep your core tight, back flat, and hips parallel to the floor. Squeeze your working-side glute to return to standing. Repeat for reps, then switch legs.

# SHOULDERS

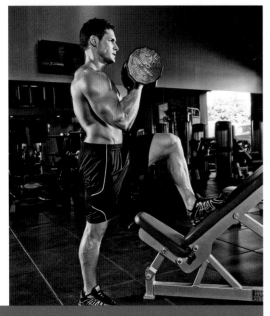

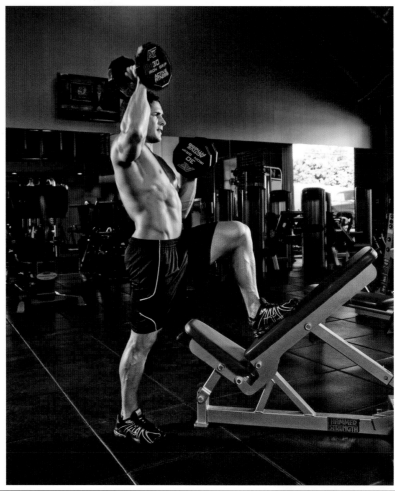

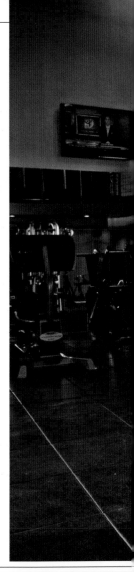

**ONE-LEG ALTERNATING ARNOLD PRESS**
>> **Start:** Set an adjustable bench to a 45-degree incline. Grasp two dumbbells at your sides and stand erect facing the bench. Place one foot on the bench's backpad so your knee is bent about 90 degrees and your center of gravity is equal between both legs. Curl the weights to shoulder level with your elbows in front of your body.
>> **Execution:** Press one dumbbell overhead as you rotate your elbow and wrist so your palm faces out at the top. Return along the same path. Alternate arms every rep and switch legs every set.

# FULL BODY

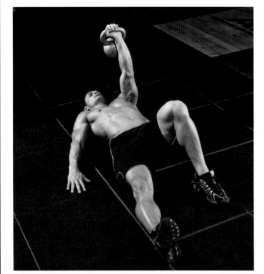

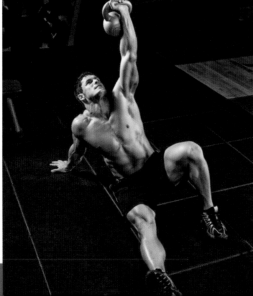

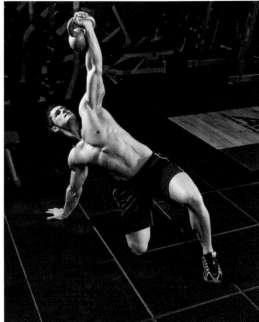

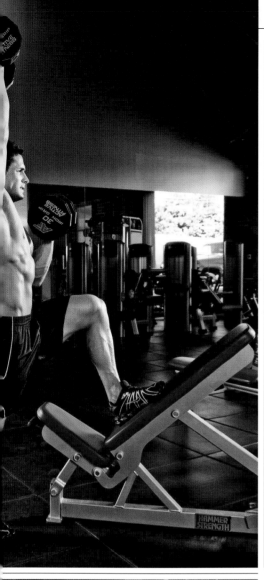

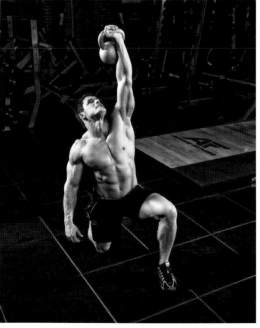

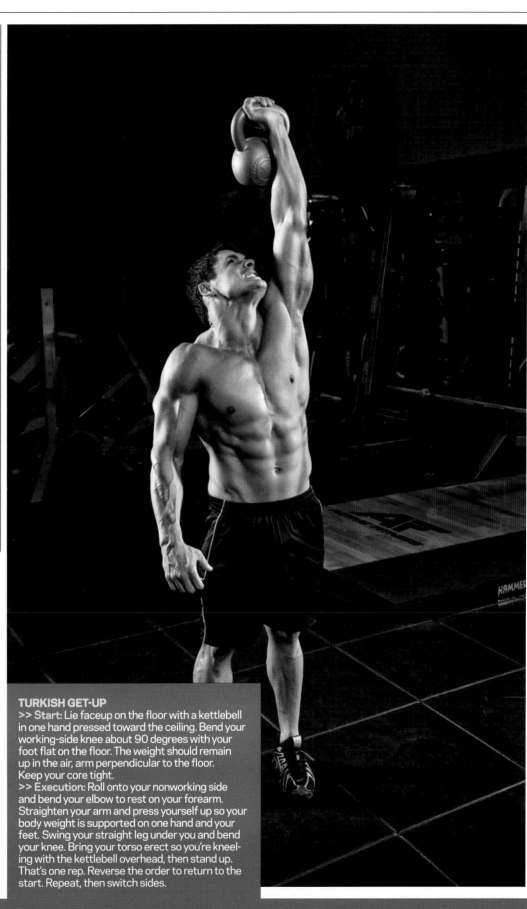

**TURKISH GET-UP**

**>> Start:** Lie faceup on the floor with a kettlebell in one hand pressed toward the ceiling. Bend your working-side knee about 90 degrees with your foot flat on the floor. The weight should remain up in the air, arm perpendicular to the floor. Keep your core tight.

**>> Execution:** Roll onto your nonworking side and bend your elbow to rest on your forearm. Straighten your arm and press yourself up so your body weight is supported on one hand and your feet. Swing your straight leg under you and bend your knee. Bring your torso erect so you're kneeling with the kettlebell overhead, then stand up. That's one rep. Reverse the order to return to the start. Repeat, then switch sides.

# SHORT CIRCUIT

## Fit in your ab workout at home with this quick yet efficient core-training program.

**A**bs are the great equalizer. If the guy next to you at the gym is a multimillionaire but his midsection looks like a pint of cookie dough that's been left in a hot car, well, the joke's on him.

"I have clients who are so smart, but they all say, 'I'm not seeing my abs. How do I get rid of this?'" demonstrates Jim Ryno, C.P.T., owner of Lift personal-training studio in Ramsey, NJ. "It comes down to how educated you are about the body. We're slowly seeing people throw in rotational and core-stabilization moves, and getting away from endless crunches."

With that in mind, Ryno has developed a short but intense abdominal circuit that can be performed almost anywhere and is designed to challenge your core on multiple levels. Two of its main components are resistance and instability. Adding these elements of difficulty not only recruits more muscle fibers but also slows you down and keeps your form honest.

"The most common mistake people make is their pace isn't steady. You see guys banging out reps and not focusing on quality," Ryno says. "They use the bounce of an exercise ball [to create momentum] instead of performing a nice, slow partial crunch. If you're doing it right and crunching at the top, you should be able to do only 15 crunches on an exercise ball, not 35."

Performing an ab workout in circuit fashion makes a lot of sense, too.

Not only does moving quickly from move to move keep boredom at bay, but it's also easy to scale a workout according to your level of conditioning. If the program isn't challenging enough, add more reps, more weight, or another exercise to the circuit. As you progress, you can perform additional circuits and/or decrease your rest time in between.

The convenience of this program makes it simple to accomplish, even on days you can't fit in your regular resistance training. While Ryno suggests doing this workout at least twice a week (preferably three), he says to let soreness be your guide. If you plan to train abs but are still doubled over from your last session, rest another day.

Yet even the most innovative workout that includes every type of rotational, resistance, and instability move imaginable can't coax your abs out of hiding if they're buried under 60 pounds of flab. Building a midsection even a millionaire would envy takes a multifaceted plan of attack.

"You need to perform high-intensity cardio, eat a clean diet, and keep your weight-training workouts at an intense level," says Ryno, who eschews isolation moves in favor of big compound exercises for getting lean. "I like recruiting as many muscle fibers as possible. I think anybody who wants abs should deadlift; biceps and triceps workouts just don't expend enough calories. If my clients want to hit biceps, we do pullups."

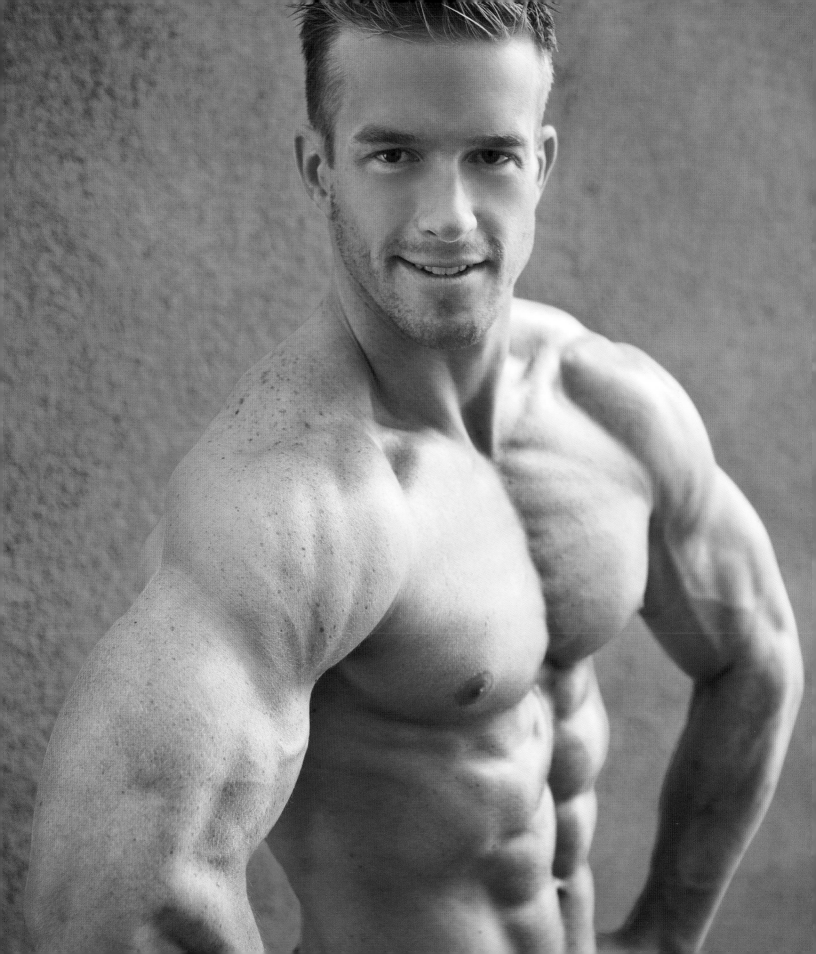

# CHAPTER 9: **SHORT CIRCUIT**

**THE PROGRAM, BY JIM RYNO, C.P.T.**
Choose three of the following five exercises and perform this routine as a circuit, moving from one exercise to the next without rest. Make sure one of the three moves utilizes the ball for stability purposes. When you finish one circuit, rest 30-90 seconds, then repeat two or three more times. Reps should range from 10-25 per exercise. Once the circuit becomes easier, increase the resistance. The abdominals are like any other muscle, so to bust through sticking points and progress you must increase the challenge. Perform this circuit at the end of your regular workout three times per week with a day of rest in between.

| EXERCISES | SETS | REPS/DISTANCE |
|---|---|---|
| Exercise-Ball Roll-Out | 2-3 | 10-25 |
| Side Plank Dumbbell Reach | 2-3 | 10-25 each side |
| Dumbbell Negative Situp | 2-3 | 10-25 |
| Side Dumbbell Crawl | 2-3 | 10 steps each |
| Exercise-Ball Dumbbell Russian Twist | 2-3 | 10 each side |

*Equipment needed: exercise ball, set of adjustable dumbbells*

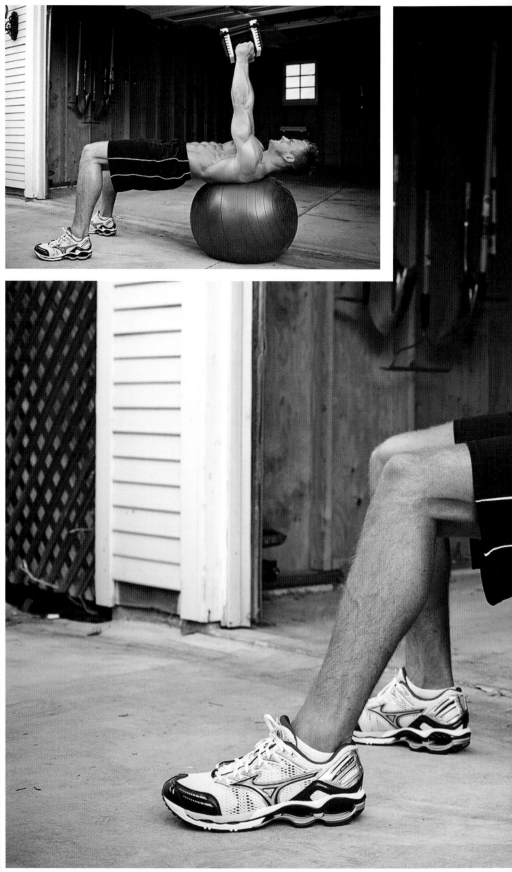

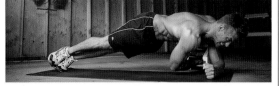

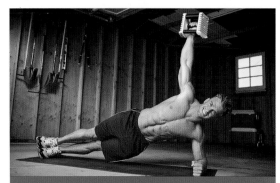

**SIDE PLANK DUMBBELL REACH**
**START:** Lie on your left side and stack your feet. Bend your left elbow 90 degrees to prop yourself up, then lift your hips off the floor until your body forms a straight line; only your left forearm and foot touch the floor. Grasp a very light dumbbell (8-10 pounds) in your right hand and extend your arm toward the ceiling.
**EXECUTION:** Slowly lower the dumbbell, and twist your hips and shoulders to bring the weight under your body and touch it to your left side. Reverse the motion to return to the start position. Make sure your left elbow is directly under your shoulder. Concentrate on keeping your hips in line with your torso; don't let them sag. Repeat for reps, then switch sides.

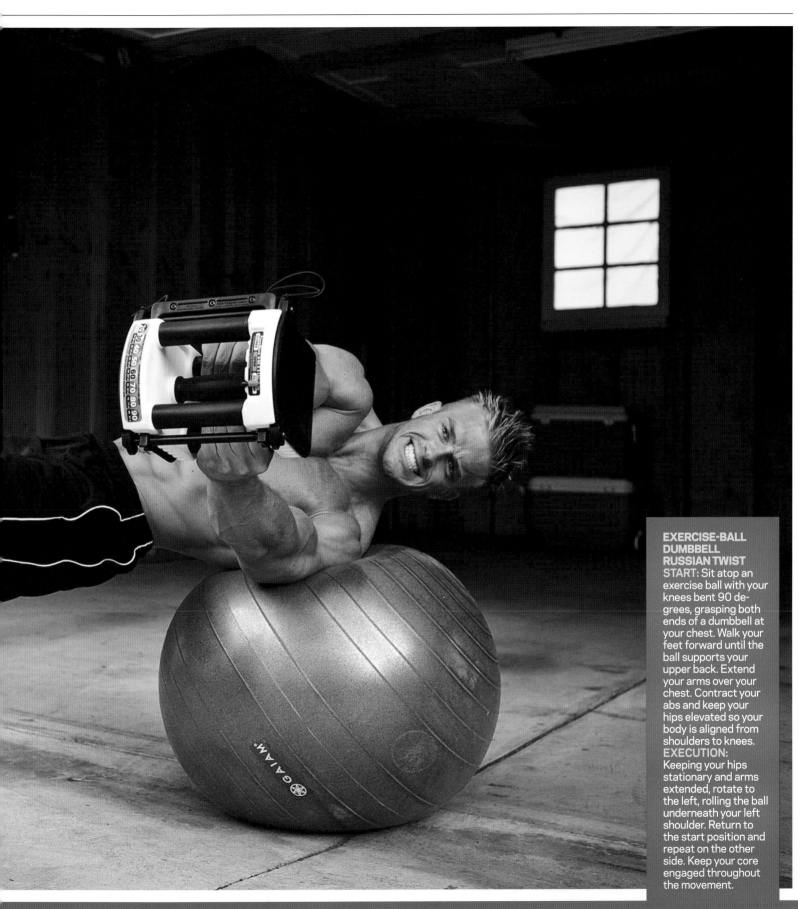

**EXERCISE-BALL DUMBBELL RUSSIAN TWIST**
**START:** Sit atop an exercise ball with your knees bent 90 degrees, grasping both ends of a dumbbell at your chest. Walk your feet forward until the ball supports your upper back. Extend your arms over your chest. Contract your abs and keep your hips elevated so your body is aligned from shoulders to knees.
**EXECUTION:** Keeping your hips stationary and arms extended, rotate to the left, rolling the ball underneath your left shoulder. Return to the start position and repeat on the other side. Keep your core engaged throughout the movement.

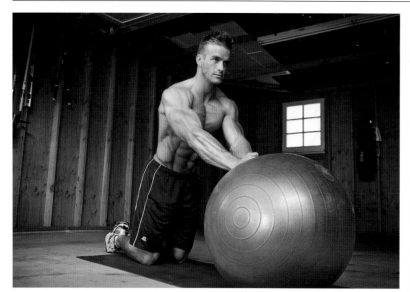

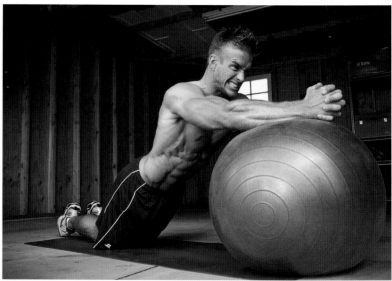

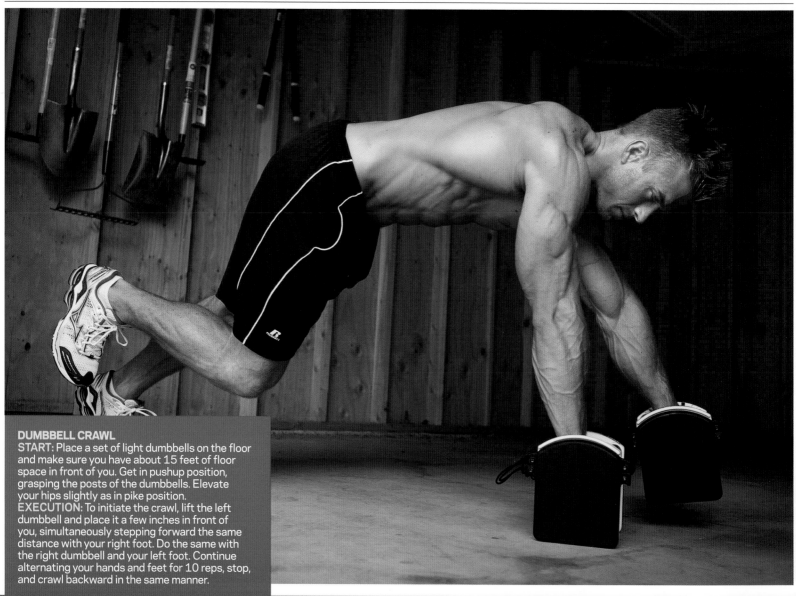

**DUMBBELL CRAWL**
**START:** Place a set of light dumbbells on the floor and make sure you have about 15 feet of floor space in front of you. Get in pushup position, grasping the posts of the dumbbells. Elevate your hips slightly as in pike position.
**EXECUTION:** To initiate the crawl, lift the left dumbbell and place it a few inches in front of you, simultaneously stepping forward the same distance with your right foot. Do the same with the right dumbbell and your left foot. Continue alternating your hands and feet for 10 reps, stop, and crawl backward in the same manner.

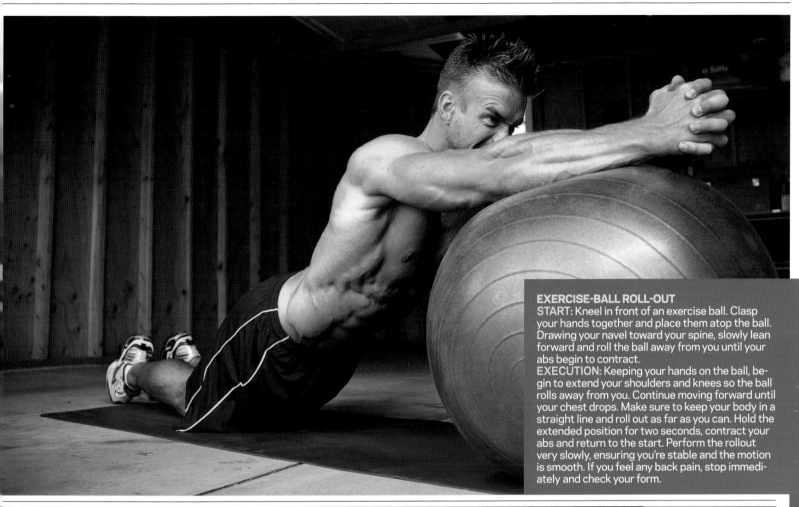

## EXERCISE-BALL ROLL-OUT

**START:** Kneel in front of an exercise ball. Clasp your hands together and place them atop the ball. Drawing your navel toward your spine, slowly lean forward and roll the ball away from you until your abs begin to contract.

**EXECUTION:** Keeping your hands on the ball, begin to extend your shoulders and knees so the ball rolls away from you. Continue moving forward until your chest drops. Make sure to keep your body in a straight line and roll out as far as you can. Hold the extended position for two seconds, contract your abs and return to the start. Perform the rollout very slowly, ensuring you're stable and the motion is smooth. If you feel any back pain, stop immediately and check your form.

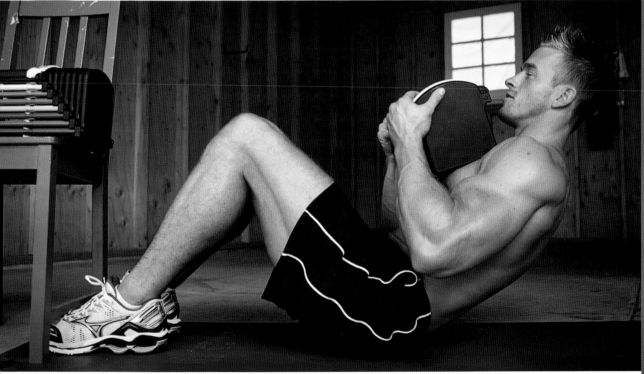

## DUMBBELL NEGATIVE SITUP

**START:** Sit on the floor with your knees bent, and your feet shoulder-width apart and hooked under a sturdy object to stabilize your body. Hold a dumbbell at your chest. Lean back slightly.

**EXECUTION:** Slowly lower your back toward the floor, keeping your abs contracted. Curl your torso forward and round your lower back as you descend. When you reach a 45-degree angle to the floor, slowly return to the start position. Make sure your abs stay tight throughout, to protect your lower back. Try to use as little momentum as possible on the return.

# [ CORE ] CONSERVATION

## Address lower-back pain and core stability with this PT-inspired ab workout.

**A**s you move through your 20s and beyond, your body's limiting factors will slowly but surely begin to emerge. This is unfortunate, but when it comes to the physical hand we humans have been dealt, it's a cold, hard fact of life. You'll feel these constraints everywhere—from the knee that buckles when the wind shifts direction to the hip flexors that won't come unbound no matter how much you stretch.

When this happens, according to Michael Camp, D.P.T., C.S.C.S., owner of Bethpage Physical Therapy in Bethpage, NY, the major keys to workout success involve recognizing these limits as they arise, accepting them as reality, and learning how best to work around them. Once you understand what you're dealing with in terms of muscular imbalances, weak points, and preexisting injuries, you can set about the work of strengthening the muscles necessary for eliminating these limiting factors for good.

In the case of direct abdominal work—the foundation of core training—this typically involves the need to both work around and attempt to fix some degree of lower-back discomfort. Whether you work a draining physical job digging ditches all day or sit at a desk pecking away on a keyboard for hours on end, back pain will eventually rear its ugly head, and it's something you'll need to address before it negatively impacts both your quality of life and the efficacy of your workouts.

"Your abs play a crucial role in everything you do," Camp says. "From general movements like getting out of a chair and walking to athletic moves such as lifting and throwing, they're the one muscle group that's constantly engaged, and it's essential to learn how to work them correctly."

When developing an ab routine you can take to the gym and perform consistently, the idea is to improve your overall core strength while minimizing—and eventually eliminating—lower-back pain as a restriction. With this in mind, the ab template Camp provides here will give you everything you need: It'll get your abs as ripped as you want while addressing the spinal stability issues that lead to various types of back pain.

"This routine is designed for anyone," he says. "The only limiting factor will be your muscular endurance, so keep the circuits in the same order, with the same movements, and just do as many reps as you can manage."

Camp strongly suggests engaging in a comprehensive cardiovascular warm-up before attempting these circuits. "You can use just about any cardio machine in the gym to warm up as long as you make sure it elevates your body temperature, increases blood flow to your muscles, and stimulates your central nervous system."

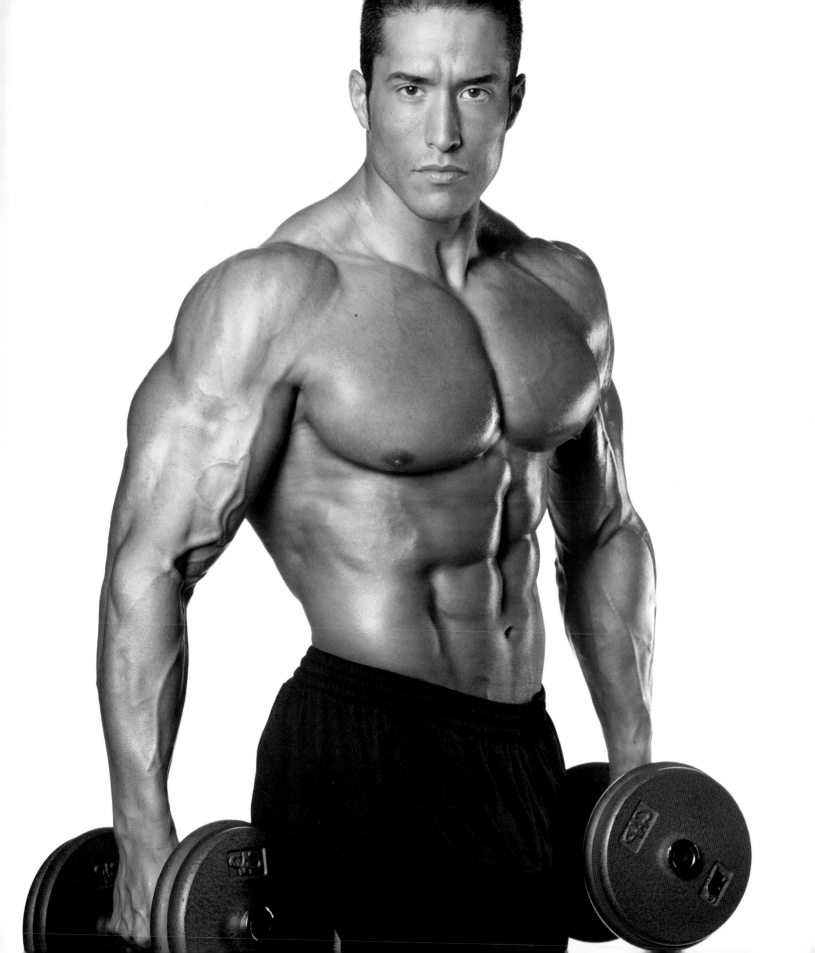

## THE ROUTINE

**Perform Camp's workout three times a week on any training day. The workout entails three circuits that combine two abdominal exercises with an active rest period. Let the "burn" factor be your guide in terms of reps. You'll be able to perform 10-50 reps depending on your experience level, so train instinctively, move from one exercise to the next with minimal rest, and repeat each circuit three times.**

| EXERCISE | REPS/TIME |
|---|---|
| **CIRCUIT 1:** | |
| Kimura Situp | To failure |
| Ab Scissor Up and Down | To failure |
| Plank* | 30 sec. |
| **CIRCUIT 2:** | |
| Thigh Slide Crunch | To failure |
| Ab Scissor Side to Side | To failure |
| Side Plank | 30 sec. |
| **CIRCUIT 3:** | |
| Straight-Leg Bicycle | To failure |
| Feet-Up Crunch and Punch | To failure |
| Side Plank | 30 sec. |

*Not pictured*

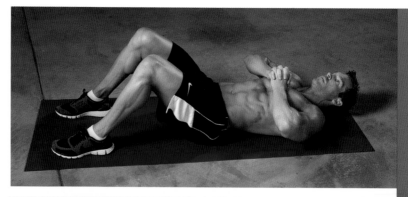

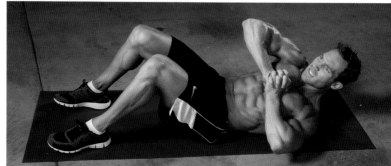

## KIMURA SITUP

**START:** Lie faceup on the floor with your hands clasped over your chest, your knees bent, and your feet flat on the floor.
**EXECUTION:** Raise your torso to approximately a 30-degree angle to the floor, then twist your shoulders slowly to bring your clasped hands to one side. Rotate back to center, lower your torso to the start position, and repeat to the other side.
**QUICK TIP:** For maximum effectiveness, keep your ab muscles contracted throughout this movement.

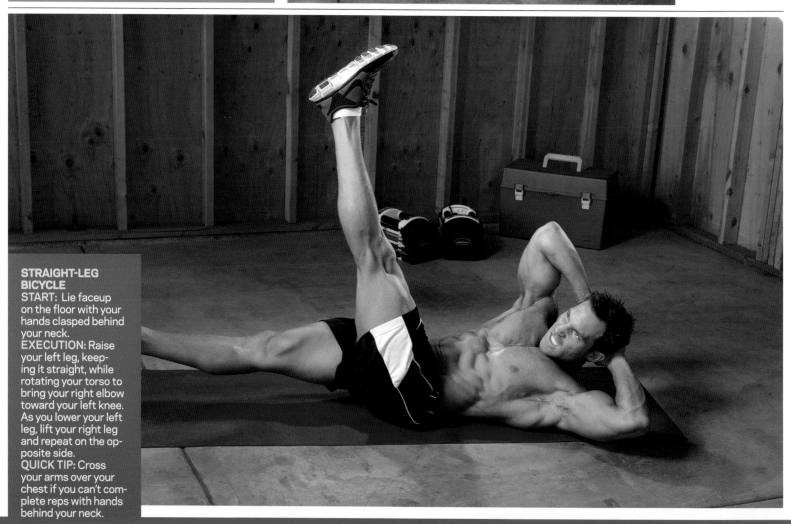

## STRAIGHT-LEG BICYCLE

**START:** Lie faceup on the floor with your hands clasped behind your neck.
**EXECUTION:** Raise your left leg, keeping it straight, while rotating your torso to bring your right elbow toward your left knee. As you lower your left leg, lift your right leg and repeat on the opposite side.
**QUICK TIP:** Cross your arms over your chest if you can't complete reps with hands behind your neck.

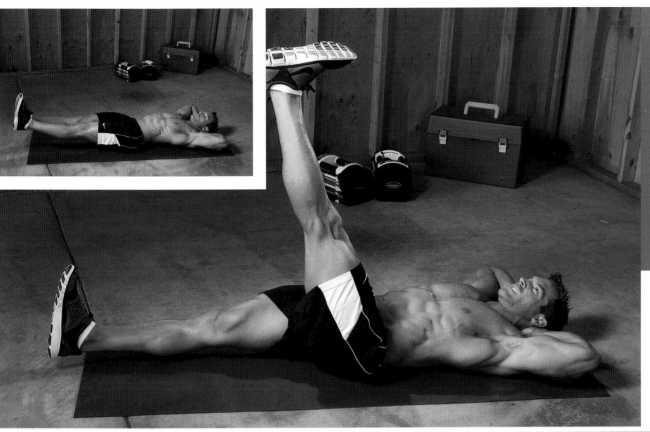

## AB SCISSOR UP AND DOWN

**START:** Lie faceup with your hands clasped behind your neck. Avoid clasping them behind your head, which can lead to neck strain.

**EXECUTION:** Keeping your legs straight, raise both feet, point your toes toward your knees, and kick your legs up and down.

**QUICK TIP:** Ab scissors are tough, but make sure you keep both feet off the floor throughout.

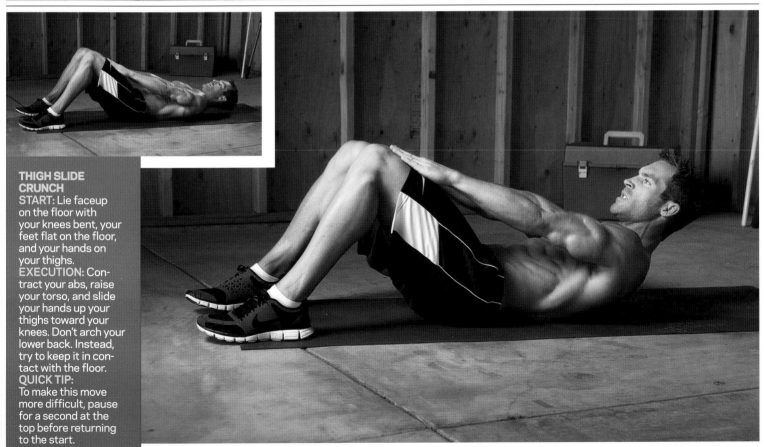

## THIGH SLIDE CRUNCH

**START:** Lie faceup on the floor with your knees bent, your feet flat on the floor, and your hands on your thighs.

**EXECUTION:** Contract your abs, raise your torso, and slide your hands up your thighs toward your knees. Don't arch your lower back. Instead, try to keep it in contact with the floor.

**QUICK TIP:** To make this move more difficult, pause for a second at the top before returning to the start.

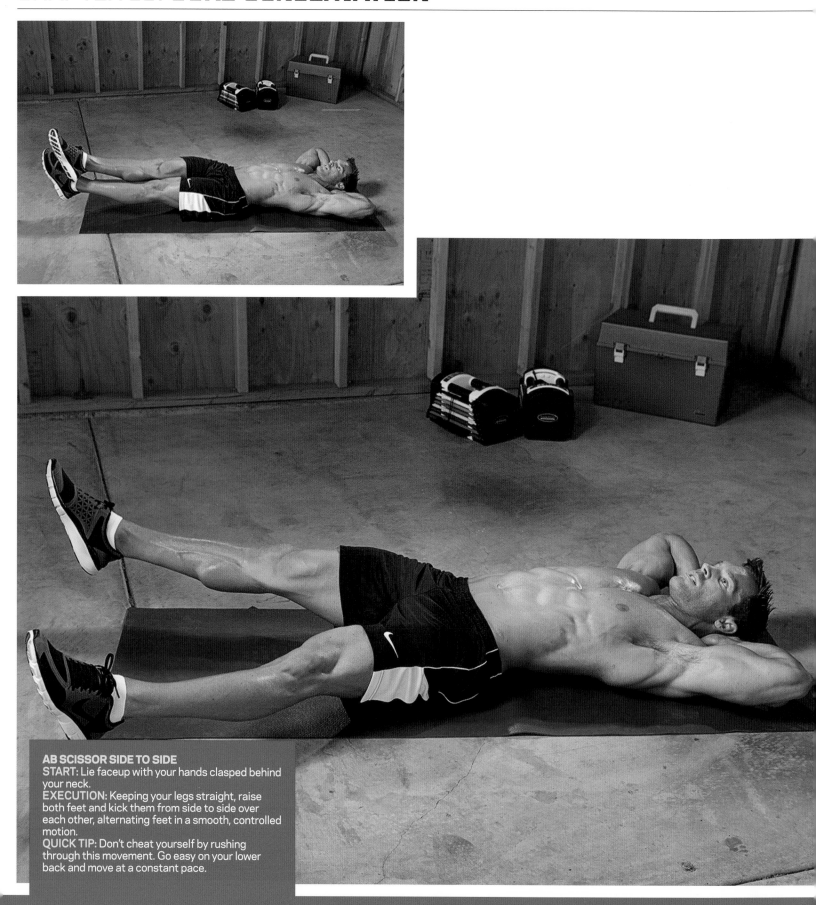

**AB SCISSOR SIDE TO SIDE**
**START:** Lie faceup with your hands clasped behind your neck.
**EXECUTION:** Keeping your legs straight, raise both feet and kick them from side to side over each other, alternating feet in a smooth, controlled motion.
**QUICK TIP:** Don't cheat yourself by rushing through this movement. Go easy on your lower back and move at a constant pace.

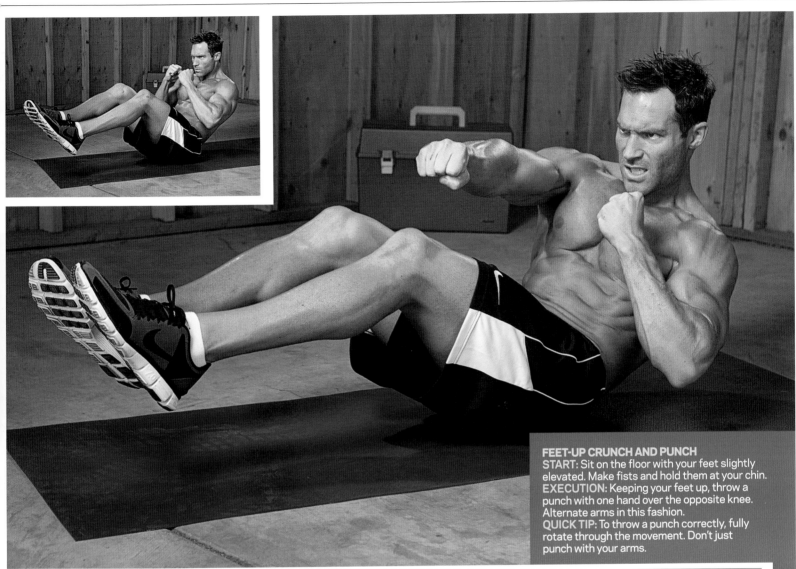

## FEET-UP CRUNCH AND PUNCH
**START:** Sit on the floor with your feet slightly elevated. Make fists and hold them at your chin.
**EXECUTION:** Keeping your feet up, throw a punch with one hand over the opposite knee. Alternate arms in this fashion.
**QUICK TIP:** To throw a punch correctly, fully rotate through the movement. Don't just punch with your arms.

## SIDE PLANK
**START:** Lie on one side with your forearm on the floor and your elbow under your shoulder.
**EXECUTION:** Push up onto your forearm, forming a straight line from head to feet. Keep your hips raised high and your shoulders and torso rotated slightly backward. Only your forearm and the side of your foot should touch the floor. Hold for 30 seconds.
**QUICK TIP:** Concentrate on keeping "body shake" to a minimum when performing any kind of plank.

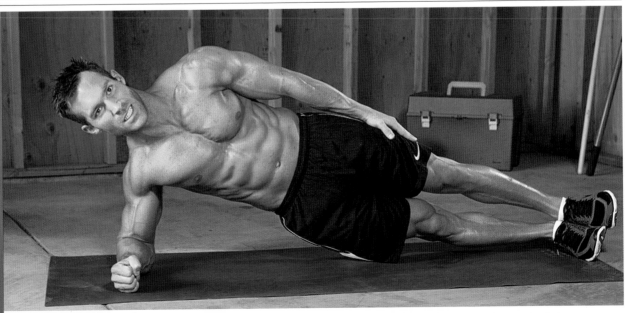

# THE FUTURE OF AB TRAINING

**Forget what you thought you knew about abs. You now hold the definitive reference guide to getting a six-pack that looks great and performs even better.**

By Alwyn Cosgrove, C.S.C.S.

**A** study came out years ago showing that certain infomercial devices activated the core better than traditional situps. What did I do? Ignored it, of course, because it was infomercial stuff. The problem was, the study appeared in the *Journal of the American Physical Therapy Association*. That's a pretty big deal. So I researched and found that all the infomercial gadgets that scored higher than the situp were basic versions of the ab-wheel rollout or the plank. Then a study came out showing that a group in the military that focused on planks and side planks outperformed a group that focused on situps—in a situp test! It became clear that various forms of stabilization, not traditional ab exercises, are the key to developing strong abs. In this chapter, I'll share what I've discovered about how your midsection really works and the way you need to train it.

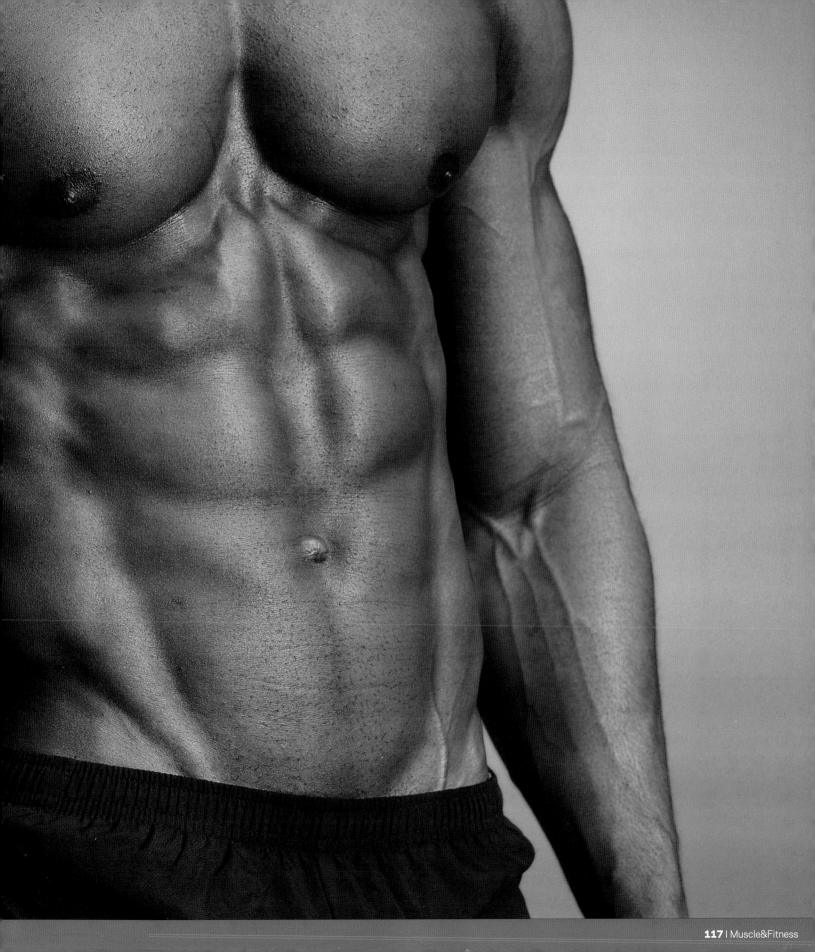

# SMARTER AB TRAINING

The primary purpose of the core—the muscles of the abdomen, including the abs, lower back, and lats—is not to flex the spine, as in crunches and situps, but to stabilize it, preventing the spine from moving. Stuart McGill, a leading expert on lower-back pain, has repeatedly shown that you can work your core more intensely with stability training than with traditional flexion exercises. It's also safer, because flexing the lumbar spine is the exact same action that can ultimately lead to disc herniation. Let me be 100% clear: I believe so strongly in training stabilization over flexion that I don't have my clients do any situp or crunch variations anymore.

At my training facility, we've further broken down core work into three distinct categories.

**Pure stabilization training.** The goal here is just to keep your spine straight, so it's as simple as holding a plank, or side plank, for time. Progressions would include elevating the feet, reducing the base of support (try raising one elbow and the opposite foot off the floor), introducing instability (such as resting your elbows on a Swiss ball), or holding for a longer time.

**Dynamic stabilization.** This is a bit of a misnomer, since dynamic means "moving" and stabilization means "don't move." But it also may best describe the true purpose of the core: to stabilize the spine while the extremities are moving. Sample exercises are a front plank with pulldown combo (get into a plank in front of a low cable pulley or resistance band, and pull the handle toward you), ab wheel rollout, mountain climber, and half-kneeling cable chop.

The goal is always to allow zero movement in the spine or core. The core muscles have to control the forces from the extremities and stabilize accordingly. With mountain climbers, for instance, there can be no lumbar flexion at all (the lower back cannot round, a common problem).

**Integrated stabilization.** This is where we do traditional exercises with a twist—for example, using one dumbbell instead of two in a lunge or shoulder press. Basically, we offset the center of gravity and force the core to work harder than it would with a traditional exercise. Sample movements would be suitcase walks (a farmer's walk, like strongmen do, but holding only one dumbbell), Turkish get-ups, and various lunges and presses with uneven loads (one heavier dumbbell in one hand or weight on one side and not the other).

That's it. Designing your core workouts with exercises that fit these categories, in my opinion, is all you'll ever need to build strong abs and an injury-resistant lower back. They can be used as a single progression—one month you could focus only on pure stabilization, work on dynamic movements the next month, and then finally do integrated stabilization exercises the month after—or as a separate focus on each of your training days. See the following sample training week to get an idea of how your core work can be scheduled. I recommend doing all core exercises, except the ones in the integrated stabilization category, first in your workouts, before you train other muscle groups.

## THE WORKOUTS

**DAY I**
**Pure Stabilization**
1 Plank
Work up to 90 seconds with feet elevated on a bench.
2 Side Plank
Work up to 45 seconds with feet elevated on a bench.

**DAY II**
**Dynamic Stabilization**
1A Sliding Disc Push-Away
10-12 reps on each arm.
–superset with–
1B Exercise-Ball Mountain Climber
10-12 reps on each leg. Rest 60 seconds and repeat the superset once more.
2 Half-kneeling Cross-Body Cable Chop
Two sets of 10-12 reps on each side.

**DAY III**
**Integrated Stabilization**
1 Turkish Get-Up Countdown
Perform five reps on each side, then four, and on down until you reach one rep. Rest only as long as you need to switch arms with the weight.
2 Suitcase Walk/Rack Walk
Walk 20 yards with the weight at your side, and then walk back with it at shoulder level. Repeat once more.

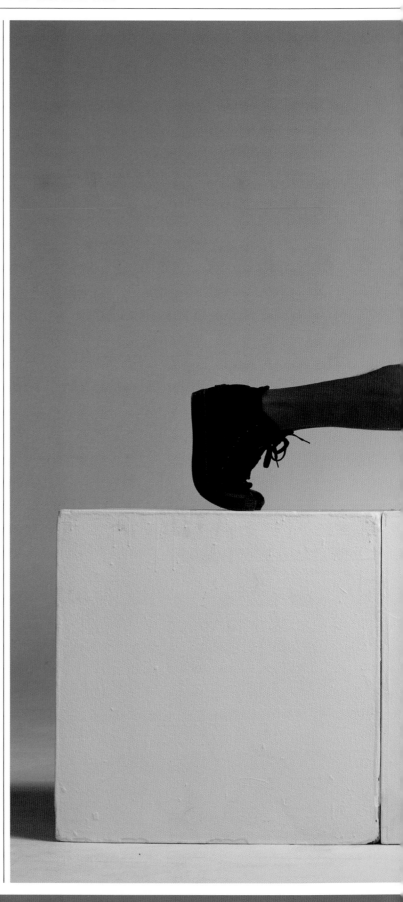

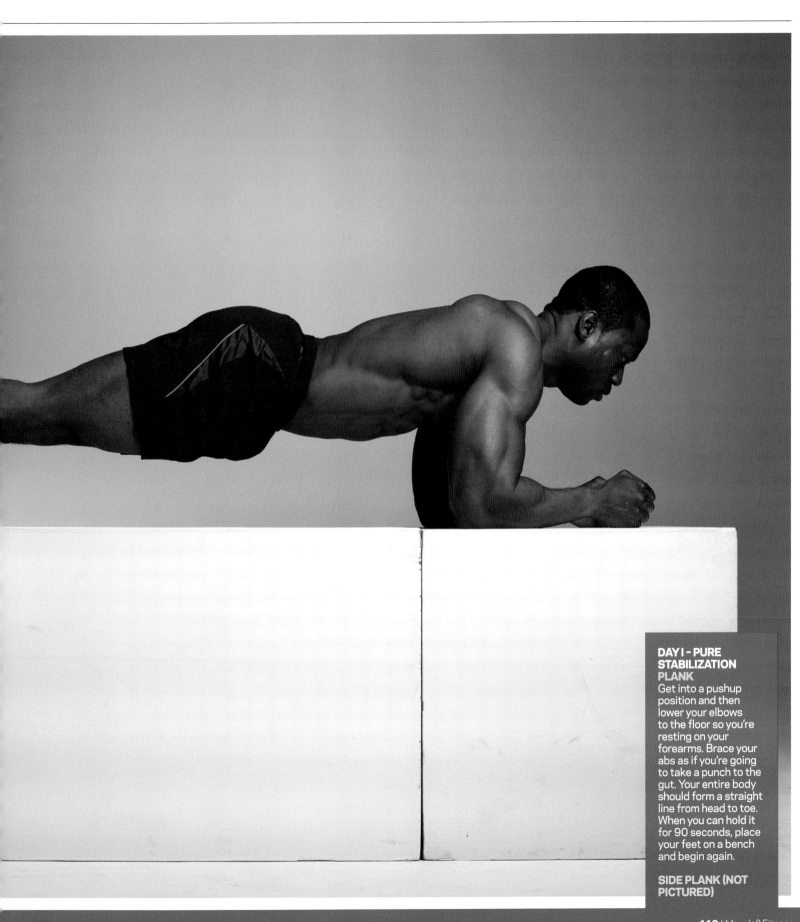

**DAY I - PURE STABILIZATION**
**PLANK**
Get into a pushup position and then lower your elbows to the floor so you're resting on your forearms. Brace your abs as if you're going to take a punch to the gut. Your entire body should form a straight line from head to toe. When you can hold it for 90 seconds, place your feet on a bench and begin again.

**SIDE PLANK (NOT PICTURED)**

HALF-KNEELING CROSS-BODY CABLE CHOP

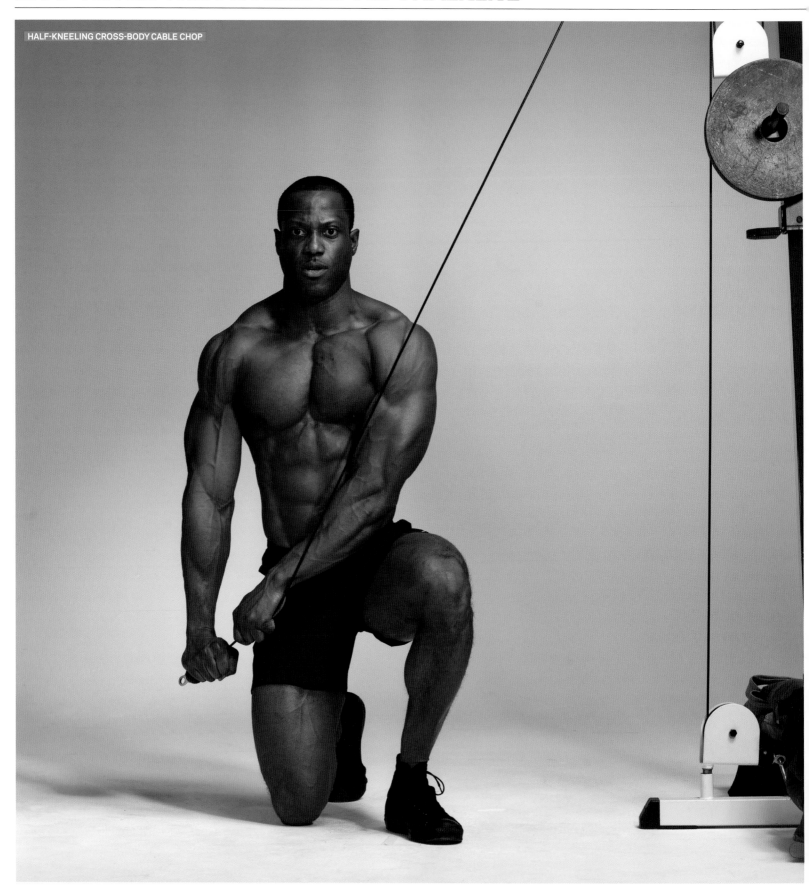

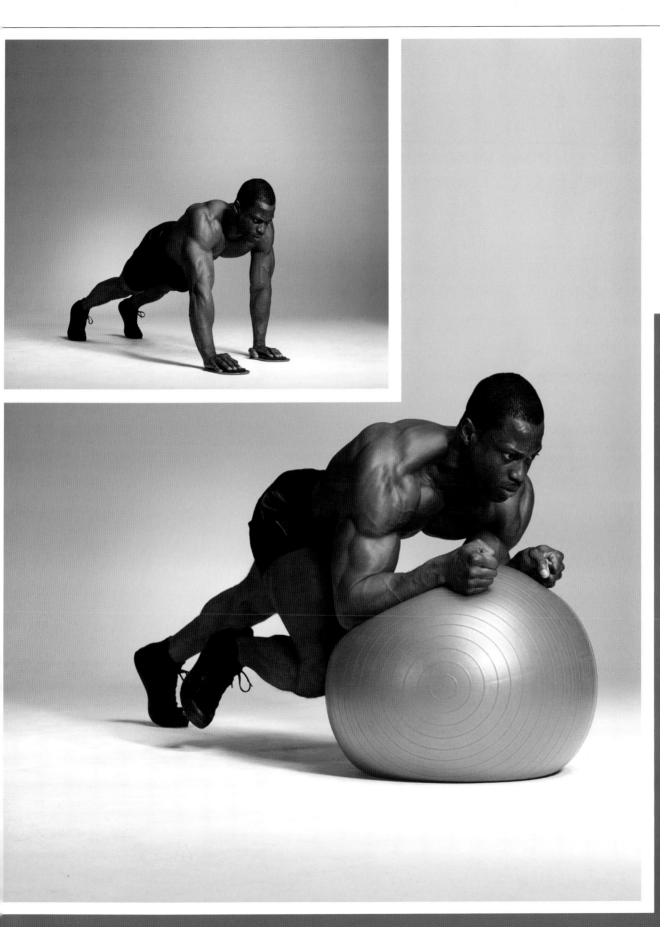

## DAY II - DYNAMIC STABILIZATION

### SLIDING DISC PUSH-AWAY
Get into a pushup position and rest each hand on a sliding disc (get a set at *valslide .com*) or weight plate wrapped in a towel. Keeping your core braced and your body in a straight line, push one arm out away from you on the floor as far as you can. Pull it back in and then repeat with the other arm.

### EXERCISE-BALL MOUNTAIN CLIMBER
Place your forearms on an exercise ball and form a straight line with your body. Brace your abs and alternately draw one knee up to the midline of your body. Lift the knee as high as you can without rounding the spine or flattening the natural curve in your lower back.

### HALF-KNEELING CROSS-BODY CABLE CHOP
Grab the bare cable from a high pulley of a cable station, and get into a lunge position next to it. Pull the cable over your left shoulder, and draw it diagonally down across your body. Do not let your torso move.

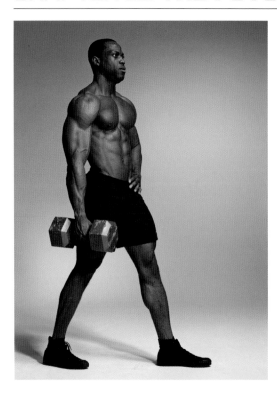

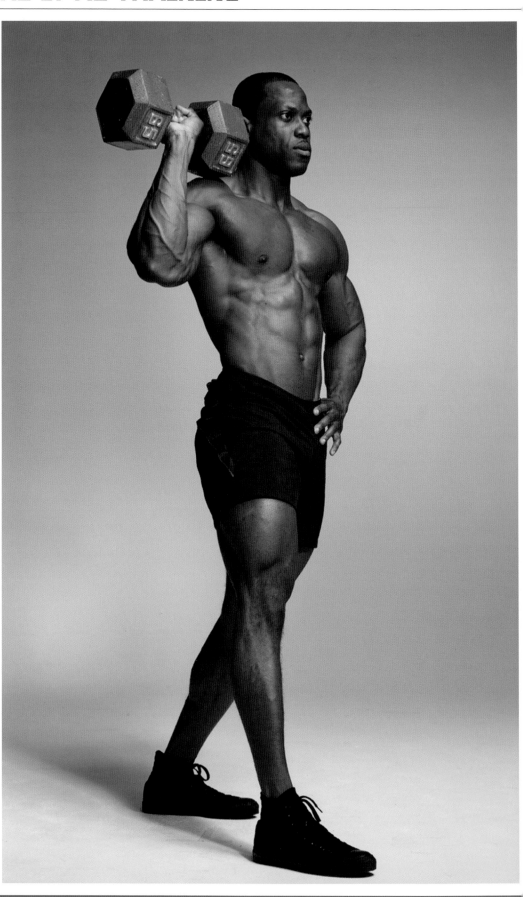

### DAY III - INTEGRATED STABILIZATION

**SUITCASE WALK/ RACK WALK**
Pick up a heavy dumbbell or kettlebell, and walk about 20 yards keeping your torso straight and the opposite hand on your hip. Now clean the weight to the rack position (shoulder height) and walk back. Repeat on the other side. Keep the opposite arm close to your side to maximize the load through your core.

**TURKISH GET-UP**
Hold a weight in your left hand and lie on the floor with your left knee bent and foot flat on the floor. Your right leg should be straight, and your right arm angled 45 degrees to your side. Now raise your torso off the floor, keeping your left arm straight overhead, and then stand up. Reverse the motion to return to the floor.

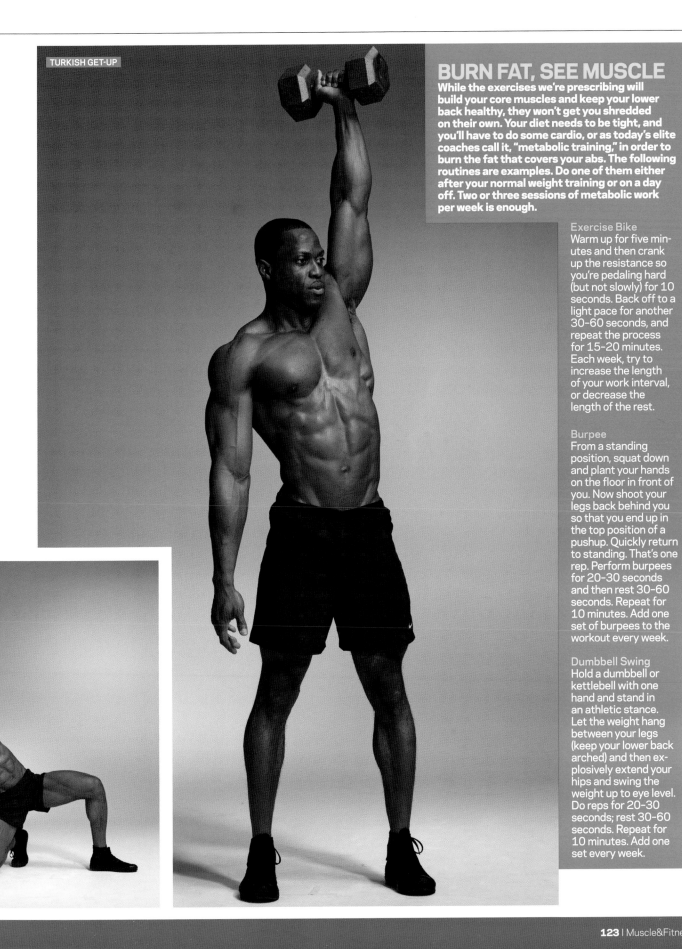

TURKISH GET-UP

# BURN FAT, SEE MUSCLE

While the exercises we're prescribing will build your core muscles and keep your lower back healthy, they won't get you shredded on their own. Your diet needs to be tight, and you'll have to do some cardio, or as today's elite coaches call it, "metabolic training," in order to burn the fat that covers your abs. The following routines are examples. Do one of them either after your normal weight training or on a day off. Two or three sessions of metabolic work per week is enough.

### Exercise Bike
Warm up for five minutes and then crank up the resistance so you're pedaling hard (but not slowly) for 10 seconds. Back off to a light pace for another 30–60 seconds, and repeat the process for 15–20 minutes. Each week, try to increase the length of your work interval, or decrease the length of the rest.

### Burpee
From a standing position, squat down and plant your hands on the floor in front of you. Now shoot your legs back behind you so that you end up in the top position of a pushup. Quickly return to standing. That's one rep. Perform burpees for 20–30 seconds and then rest 30–60 seconds. Repeat for 10 minutes. Add one set of burpees to the workout every week.

### Dumbbell Swing
Hold a dumbbell or kettlebell with one hand and stand in an athletic stance. Let the weight hang between your legs (keep your lower back arched) and then explosively extend your hips and swing the weight up to eye level. Do reps for 20–30 seconds; rest 30–60 seconds. Repeat for 10 minutes. Add one set every week.

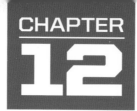

# FAST-FORWARD YOUR FAT LOSS

**Serious about getting lean sooner rather than later? This super-charged program combines lifting and cardio to melt away pounds of body fat in just four weeks.**

It takes a combination of efforts to get lean to achieve a better six-pack. You have to eat right and train hard, not just one or the other. And when it comes to the latter, you need a solid lifting plan and cardio regimen. Just hitting the weights isn't enough, and simply plodding away on a treadmill will for the most part leave you spinning your fat-loss wheels. The following program is truly a synthesis, bringing together high-volume lifting and super-intense cardio: It's a mix of high- and low-rep training plus interval-based cardio and longer, steady-state exercise. That's because one without the other might have you burning some body fat, but not nearly as much as you're capable of. Over the next four weeks, the workouts will be tough and the month might seem long, but at the end of the program you'll surely realize why you did it. You'll have burned lots of blubber and your abs will be showing. Not a bad combination, huh?

The program has you train six days a week (Monday through Saturday), each workout consisting of both lifting weights and cardio. You'll do more or less the same routines every week, and due to the high volume and intense nature of the workouts, this plan will be very effective since your body will still be adapting to the stress placed on it through the fourth week. Here's a general rundown of what each day will entail.

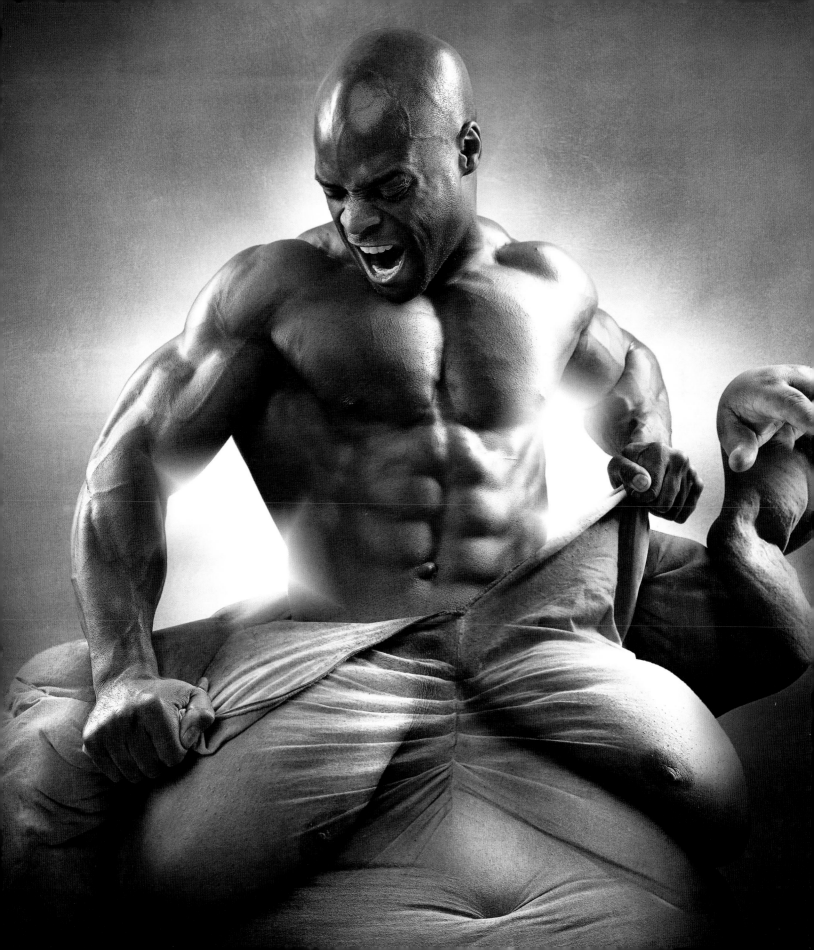

## DAY 1 | MONDAY

The training week will start with a high-volume arm workout and a heavy-duty cardio session, performed in that order. The weightlifting will consist of three exercises each for biceps and triceps.

For biceps, start off with what's called a buddy curl. First, select a weight with which you'll reach failure at around 10 reps. Do one rep, then pass the bar to your training partner. He'll do his rep, then hand the bar back to you for two reps. Hand it back to him for two reps, then it's back to you for three reps, and so on. Do this in one-rep increments until you reach 10 reps on your last set. (If you don't have a lifting partner, set the bar down on a bench between sets and rest as long as it would take someone else to do the same number of reps.) This method is great for adding volume and intensity to your workout, which are hallmarks of this program. Perform all the other exercises for biceps and triceps in straight-set fashion.

As you'll notice, nearly every exercise (one exception being buddy curls) will consist of three to four sets of reps ranging from 6–20. Go heavy on your first set to hit the low end of this range, then progressively lighten the load so you're doing 20 reps by your third or fourth set. This makes your muscles work with heavy, moderate, and light weights, all in the span of minutes for each exercise, which keeps your body guessing and less likely to adapt to a constant resistance. Moreover, the heavy sets help you maintain muscle in the midst of the clean dieting and extensive cardio you'll undertake, both of which can strip away muscle along with the fat if you're not careful.

The cardio routine planned for Mondays will be repeated on Thursday and Friday each week, and it represents the most intense sessions you'll do over the course of the program. It consists of three elements: 1) one-minute intervals of jumping rope, 2) 30-second intervals using a heavy rope, and 3) 50 reps of bench jumps, 25 to each side of the bench. Perform this circuit 10 times through for an intense cardio workout that'll melt away body fat. Each week, increase the volume of each move: Add a minute to each jump rope interval, 30 seconds to each heavy rope bout, and 10 reps to each set of bench jumps.

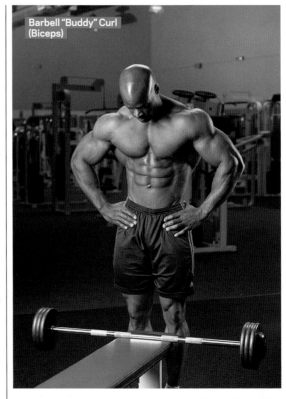

Barbell "Buddy" Curl (Biceps)

### INTENSIVE FAT-LOSS TRAINING SPLIT

| DAY | BODY PART(S) TRAINED |
|---|---|
| 1 | Arms, Cardio (intense) |
| 2 | Legs, Cardio (easy) |
| 3 | Cardio (easy, long), Abs, Calves |
| 4 | Chest, Shoulders, Cardio (intense) |
| 5 | Back, Traps, Cardio (intense) |
| 6 | Cardio (easy, long), Abs, Calves |
| 7 | Rest |

### DAY 1 | ARMS

| EXERCISE | SETS | REPS |
|---|---|---|
| **BICEPS** | | |
| Barbell "Buddy" Curl | 2 | 55[1] |
| Incline Cable Curl | 3-4 | 6-20 |
| Dumbbell Preacher Curl | 3-4 | 6-20 |
| **TRICEPS** | | |
| Weighted Bench Dip | 3-4 | 6-20 |
| Triceps Pressdown | 3-4 | 6-20 |
| Standing Overhead Cable Extension | 3-4 | 6-20 |

[1]*Select a weight that causes you to fail at around 10 reps. Do one rep, then rest one second or as long as it takes your partner to do one rep. Then do two reps, resting as long as it takes your partner to do two reps, and so on until you've reached 10 reps. That's one set.*

### CARDIO

| EXERCISE | DURATION/REPS |
|---|---|
| Jump Rope | 1 minute |
| Heavy Rope | 30 seconds |
| Bench Jump | 25 reps* |

>> *Perform these exercises as a circuit 10 times.*
>> *During Weeks 2-4, increase your jump-rope time by one minute each week, increase the heavy rope time by 30 seconds and increase your bench jumps by 10 reps. By Week 4, you should be doing four minutes of jumping rope, two minutes of heavy rope, and 55 reps of bench jumps per circuit.*
*Jumping over the bench and back is one rep.*

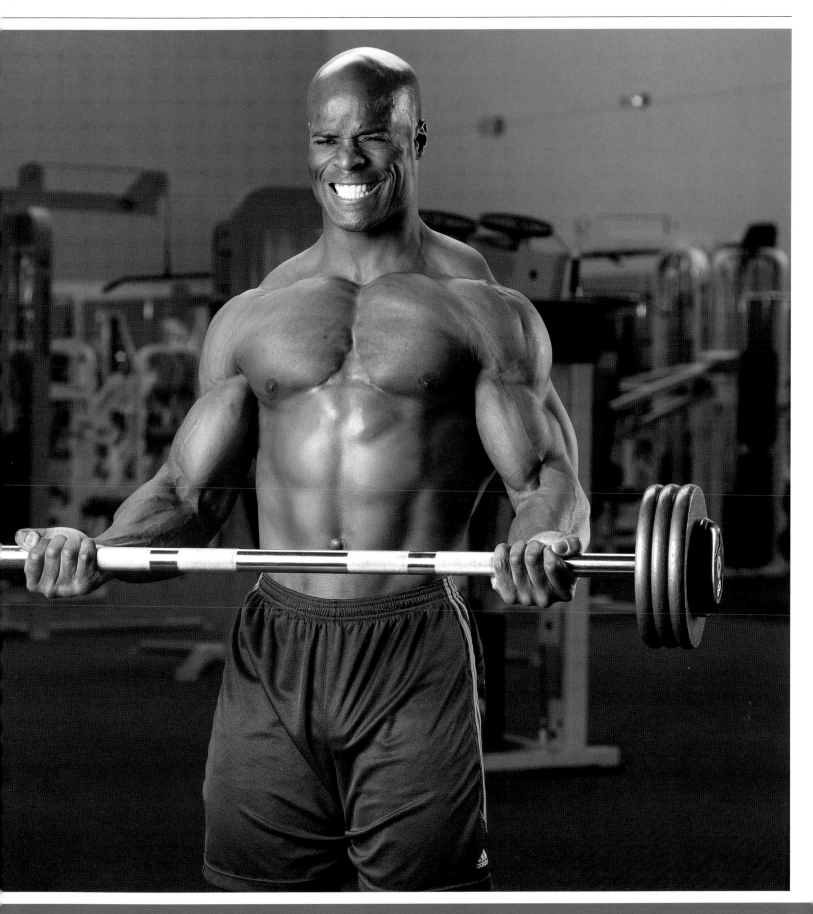

## DAY 2 | TUESDAY

Your second session of the week is leg day. And we'll be honest: It's high-volume, very intense work. The workout consists of basic compound exercises, such as squats and leg presses, and three different supersets to hit the largest muscles of the lower body—the quads, glutes, and hamstrings. A couple of novel exercises, the barbell crawl and jump squat, are thrown in to provide a further shock to the body.

Because your legs will no doubt be thoroughly exhausted after performing 10 total movements for the lower body, you'll do a relatively easy cardio session immediately afterward. Again, you'll jump rope, but this time alternate jumping for one minute at an easy pace with resting one minute for 40 minutes. Think of it this way: You'll actually be jumping rope for only 20 minutes.

### DAY 2 | LEGS

| EXERCISE | SETS | REPS |
|---|---|---|
| Barbell Squat | 3-4 | 6-20 |
| — superset with — | | |
| Barbell Crawl[1] | 3-4 | 40- to 60-foot walk |
| Leg Press | 3-4 | 6-20 |
| Leg Extension | 3-4 | 6-20 |
| — superset with — | | |
| Jump Squat | 3-4 | 6-20 |
| Romanian Deadlift | 3-4 | 6-20 |
| Lying Leg Curl | 3-4 | 6-20 |
| — superset with — | | |
| Body-Weight Jump Squat | 3-4 | 20 |

[1]*Immediately after each set of squats, place a short, empty bar across your back, squat down, and walk approximately 20–30 feet. Then stop, turn around, and return to your starting point.*

**CARDIO**
*Jump Rope: 1 minute on, 1 minute off for 40 minutes (this totals 20 minutes of jumping rope and 20 minutes of rest)*

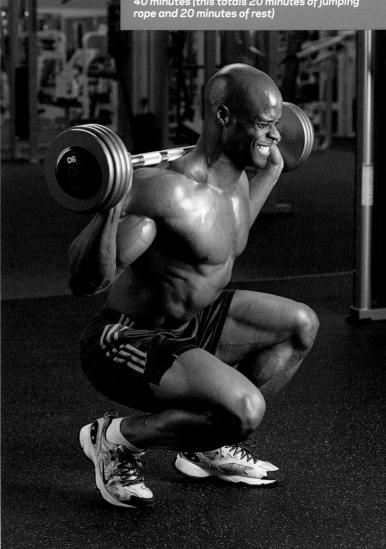

Barbell Crawl (Legs)

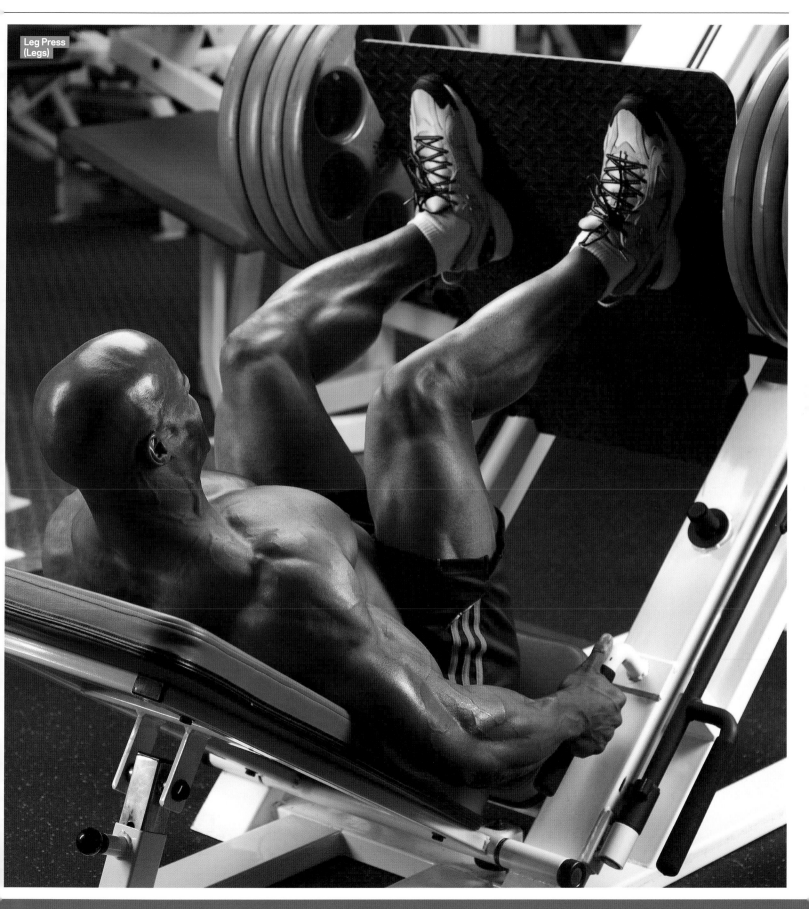

# DAYS 3 & 6 |
# WEDNESDAY & SATURDAY

These two days are identical during all four weeks of the program. Each time, perform cardio first, followed by a short ab and calves workout. The cardio session (either a walk on a treadmill or stair-stepper) will be low in intensity and long—two hours long, to be exact. This serves as a drastic change of pace from the high-intensity cardio work you do on Monday, Thursday, and Friday, and that's just the point. Your body will burn more fat by training at both high and low intensities.

The lifting on these days will be minimal, only abs and calves with six sets total for each. Feel free to keep your rest periods short between sets (30–45 seconds) to move the workout along quickly.

**DAY 3 | ABS + CALVES**
**CARDIO**
*Treadmill or stair-stepper: Two hours at low intensity (50%–60% of max heart rate)*

| EXERCISE | SETS | REPS |
| --- | --- | --- |
| **ABS** | | |
| Hanging Leg Raise | 3 | To failure |
| Machine Crunch | 3 | 10-12 |
| **CALVES** | | |
| Standing Calf Raise | 3 | 20 |
| Seated Calf Raise | 3 | 20 |

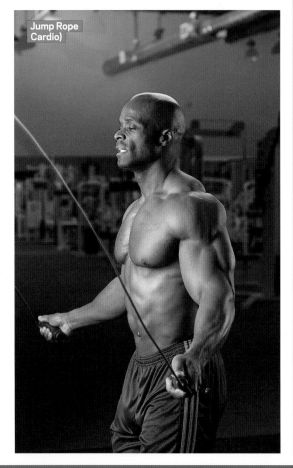

Jump Rope (Cardio)

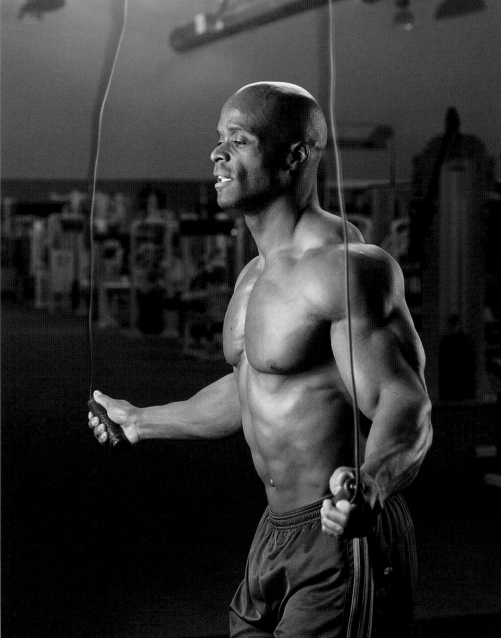

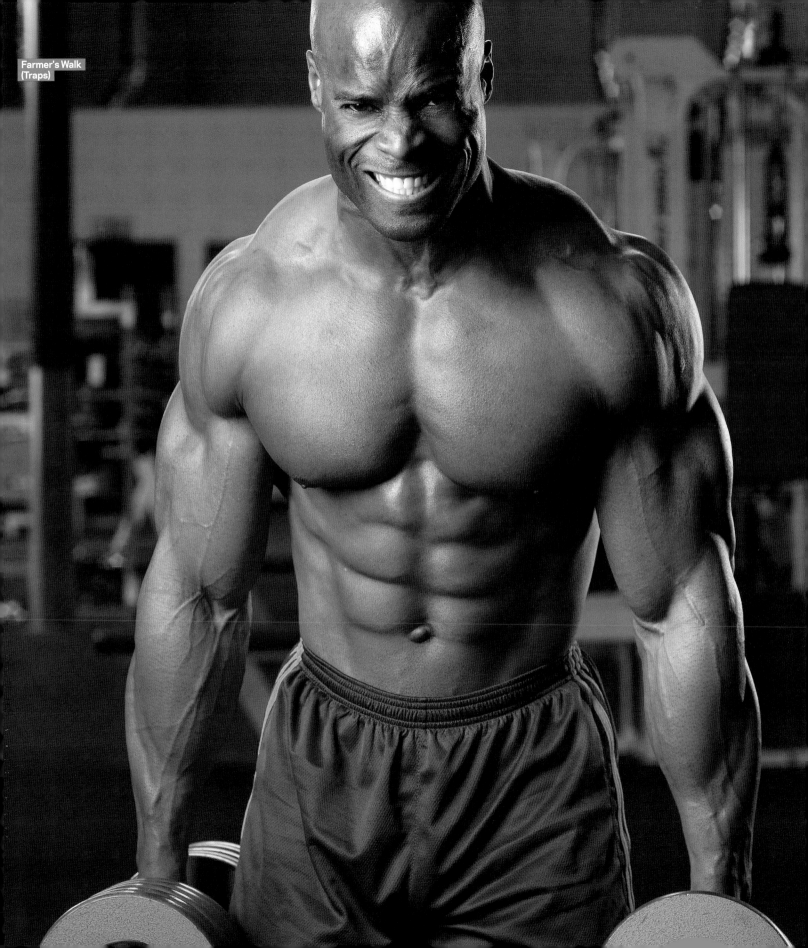

# DAY 4 | THURSDAY

Chest and shoulders are on tap for Thursdays, followed by the same cardio workout you did on Monday. The exercises for pecs and delts are mostly basic, compound movements to hit the most muscle fibers possible to maximize calorie-burning. The volume is elevated (five exercises for chest, three for shoulders) to burn more calories during the workout and keep your metabolism elevated afterward.

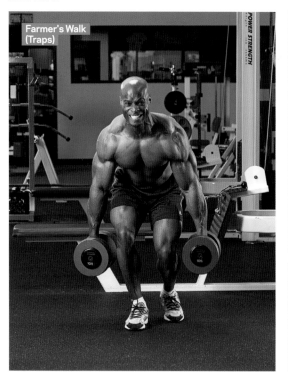

Farmer's Walk (Traps)

| DAY 4 | CHEST + SHOULDERS | | |
|---|---|---|
| EXERCISE | SETS | REPS |
| **CHEST** | | |
| Incline Dumbbell Press | 3-4 | 6-20 |
| Incline Dumbbell Flye | 3-4 | 6-20 |
| Bench Press | 3-4 | 6-20 |
| Pec-Deck Flye | 3-4 | 6-20 |
| Smith Machine Decline Press | 3-4 | 6-20 |
| **SHOULDERS** | | |
| Overhead Dumbbell Press | 3-4 | 6-20 |
| Cable Lateral Raise | 3-4 | 6-20 |
| Bentover Cable Lateral Raise | 3-4 | 6-20 |

| CARDIO | |
|---|---|
| EXERCISE | DURATION/REPS |
| Jump Rope | 1 minute |
| Heavy Rope | 30 seconds |
| Bench Jump | 25 reps* |

>> *Perform these exercises as a circuit 10 times.*
>> *During Weeks 2-4, increase your jump rope time by one minute each week, increase the heavy rope time by 30 seconds, and increase your bench jumps by 10 reps. By Week 4, you should be doing four minutes of jumping rope, two minutes of heavy rope, and 55 reps of bench jumps per circuit.*
*Jumping over the bench and back is one rep.*

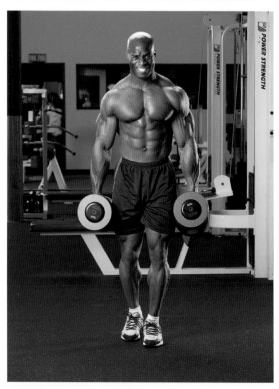

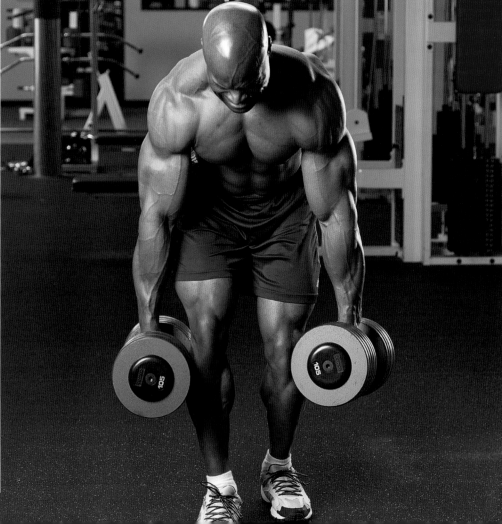

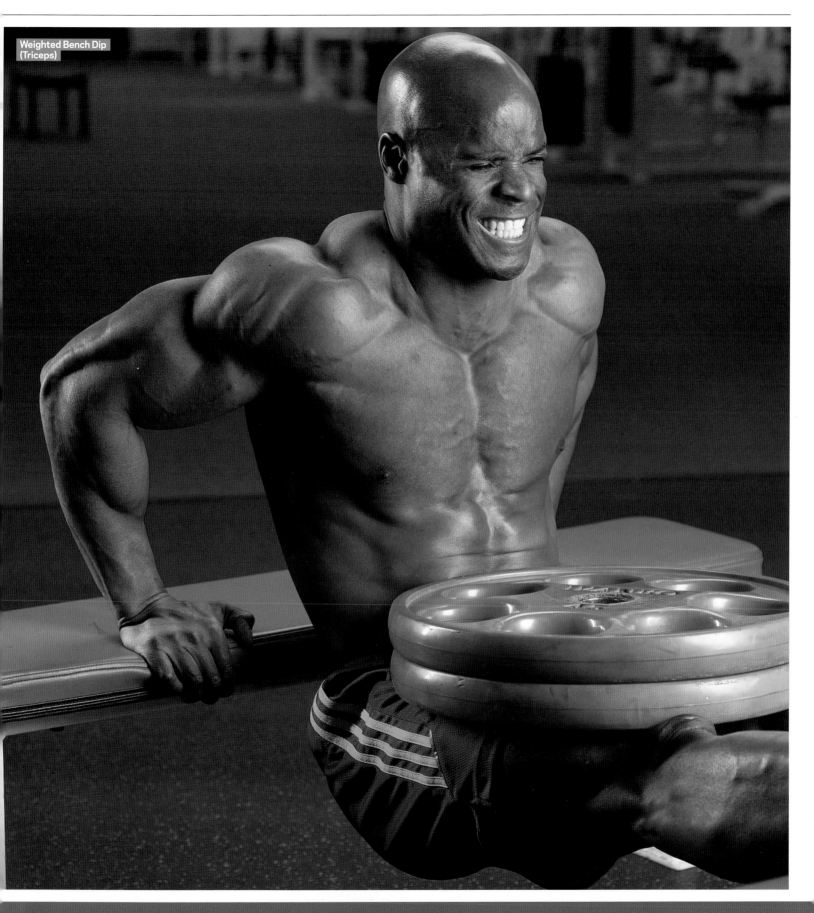

Weighted Bench Dip
(Triceps)

## DAY 5 | FRIDAY

Back and traps are the focus on Fridays, followed by the jump rope/bench jump cardio routine from Monday and Thursday. Train your back with high volume (four exercises) and fundamental exercises such as dumbbell deadlifts and T-bar rows.

For traps, in addition to dumbbell shrugs, you'll do the strongman exercise known as the farmer's walk. This is considered a trap exercise because the upper traps will likely be the first muscles to succumb to exhaustion. (To ensure that your hands and forearms don't go first, you may want to use wrist straps.) But make no mistake, the farmer's walk involves myriad other muscles, from the upper back to the legs, making it a great calorie burner that's ideal for this program.

And there you have it—the perfect combination of no-nonsense lifting and fat-blasting cardio. For the next four weeks, you'll subject your body to a multitude of training intensities and durations—the best of both worlds. Get ready to get lean in a hurry.

### DAY 5 | BACK + TRAPS

| EXERCISE | SETS | REPS |
|---|---|---|
| **BACK** | | |
| Dumbbell Deadlift | 3-4 | 6-20 |
| T-Bar Row | 3-4 | 6-20 |
| Straight-Arm Lat Pulldown | 3-4 | 6-20 |
| Seated Row | 3-4 | 6-20 |
| **TRAPS** | | |
| Farmer's Walk [1] | 3-4 | To failure |
| Dumbbell Shrug | 3-4 | 6-20 |

[1] *Select a weight that matches your 8- to 10-rep max on dumbbell shrugs (a relatively heavy weight). Hold the weights at your sides and walk approximately 20-30 feet. Stop, turn around, and return to the start. Continue until you can no longer hold on to the weights due to upper-trap fatigue.*

### CARDIO

| EXERCISE | DURATION/REPS |
|---|---|
| Jump Rope | 1 minute |
| Heavy Rope | 30 seconds |
| Bench Jump | 25 reps* |

*>> Perform these exercises as a circuit 10 times.*
*>> During Weeks 2-4, increase your jump-rope time by one minute each week, increase the heavy rope time by 30 seconds, and increase your bench jumps by 10 reps. By Week 4, you should be doing four minutes of jumping rope, two minutes of heavy rope, and 55 reps of bench jumps per circuit.*
*\*Jumping over the bench and back is one rep.*

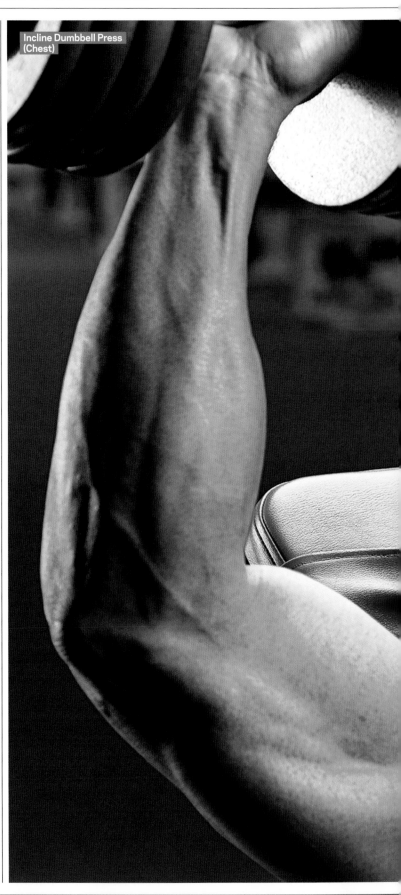

Incline Dumbbell Press (Chest)

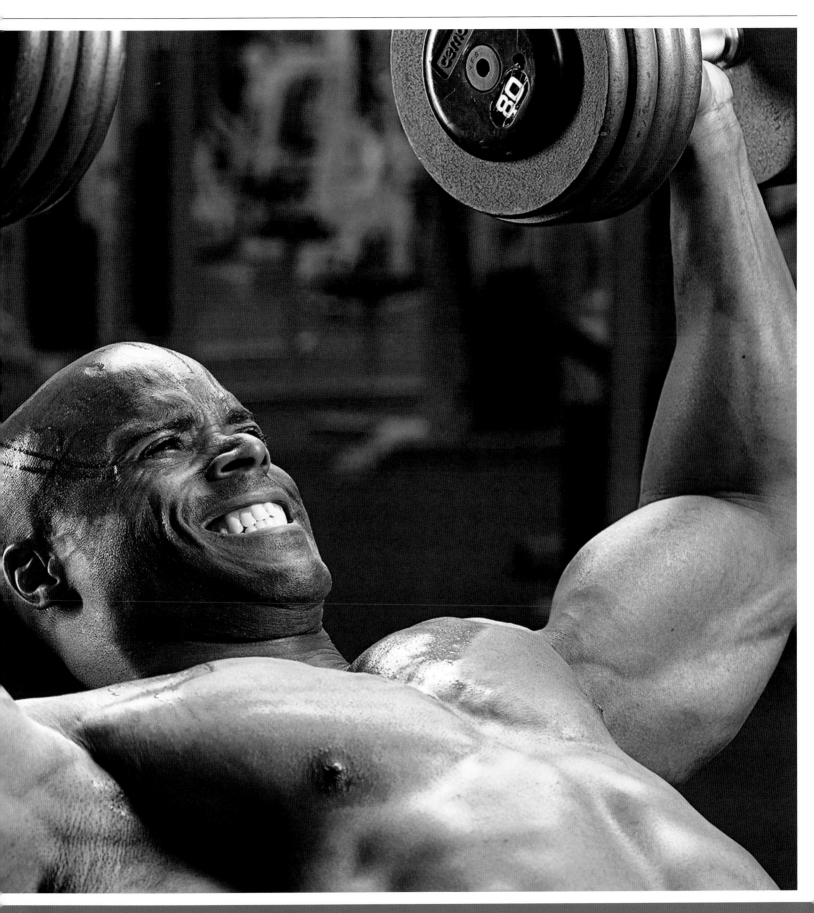

**DAY 6 I ABS + CALVES**
**CARDIO**
*Treadmill or stair-stepper: Two hours at a low intensity (50%-60% of max heart rate)*

| EXERCISE | SETS | REPS |
|---|---|---|
| **ABS** | | |
| Hanging Leg Raise | 3 | To failure |
| Machine Crunch | 3 | 10-12 |
| **CALVES** | | |
| Standing Calf Raise | 3 | 20 |
| Seated Calf Raise | 3 | 20 |

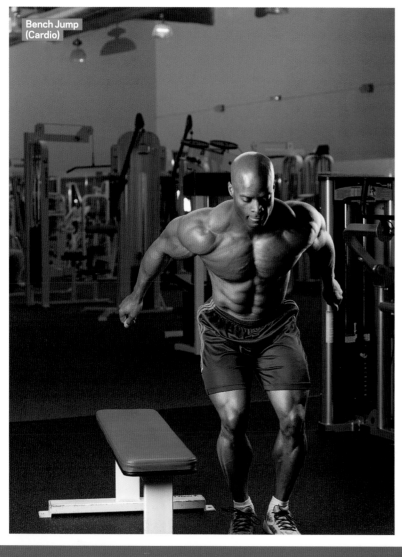

Bench Jump
(Cardio)

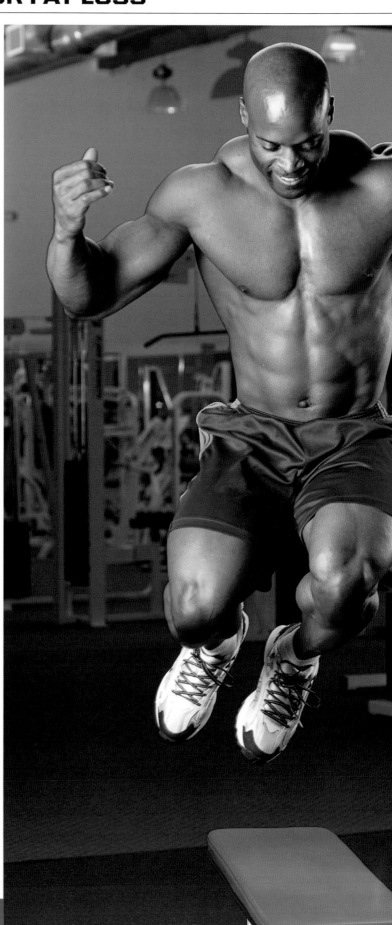

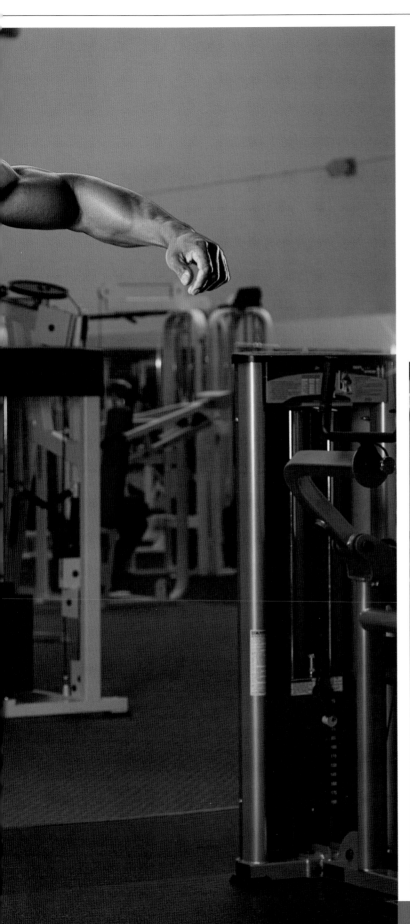

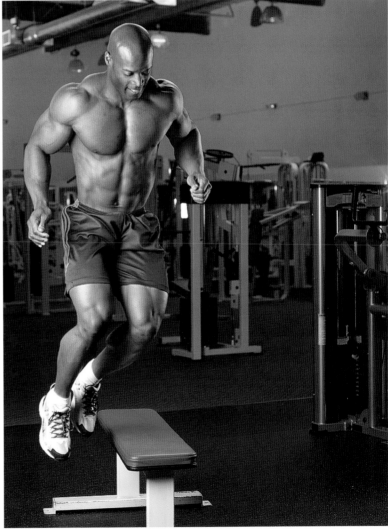

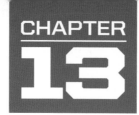

# KILLER COMBOS

## How to use supersets, trisets, and giant sets to speed up your workouts and burn more body fat for better abs.

I f you spend 90 minutes in the gym every day in your quest to build muscle, burn fat, and get a better six-pack, surely you'd get only half the benefit if you worked out for just 45 minutes, right? After all, it takes ample time to train fairly heavy, sufficiently rest between sets, perform several sets per exercise, hit the muscles from all angles, and train multiple body parts. You figure that anything that shortchanges your workout also shortchanges the results. Wrong. Doing supersets—combining exercises in back-to-back fashion without resting in between—has long been a tool among the lunchtime crowd looking to get in shape in a limited amount of time.

Competitive bodybuilders have incorporated the concept of doing successive exercises with no rest in between for decades to increase muscle definition and burn calories, which also translates into a leaner midsetion. This high-intensity technique isn't meant to be followed indefinitely, but it can be used to shake up your training or even just speed things up on days when you simply want a fast workout.

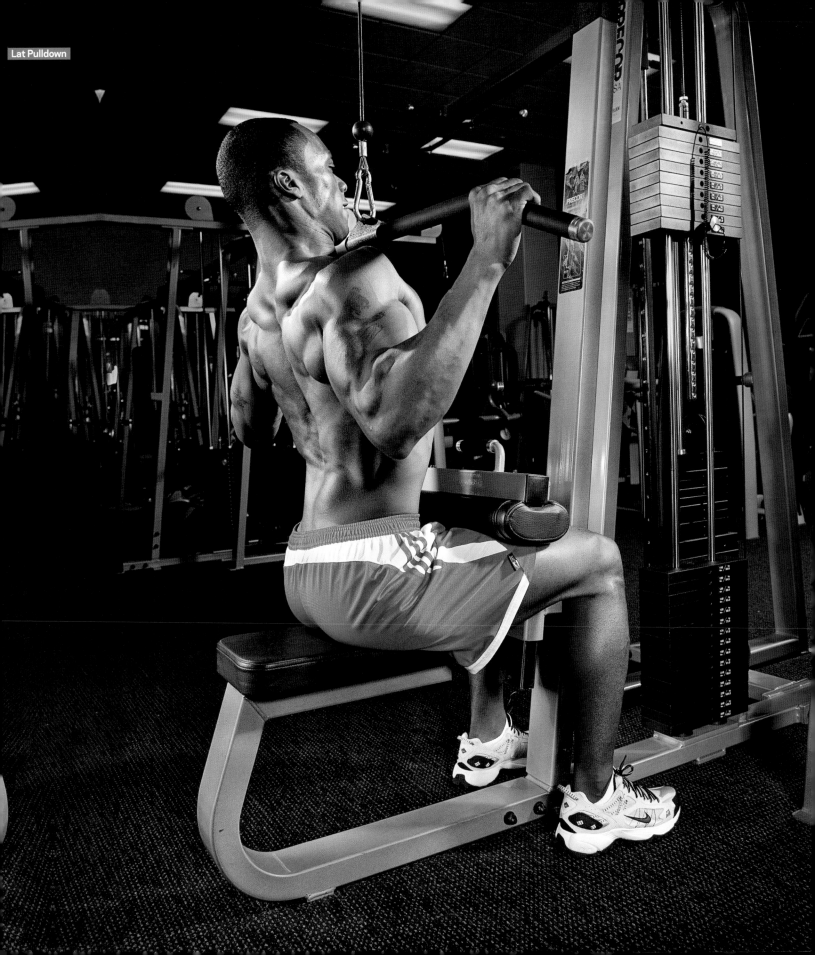

# LINKING MOVES

The difference between supersets, trisets, and giant sets relates to the number of exercises you perform consecutively before resting.

>> A superset consists of two exercises performed back to back with no rest in between. Rest only after you complete both moves. A superset can include exercises that work opposing muscles (such as biceps and triceps) or the same muscle group (sometimes called a compound set). You can think of a superset as one long set with two different moves; the only requirement is that you keep rest to an absolute minimum, only as long as it takes to go from one exercise to the next in the shortest possible time.

Antagonist (opposing) muscle groups, which work around the same joint(s), include the following: triceps/biceps, quads/hamstrings, chest/back, abs/ lower back, and forearm flexors/wrist extensors.

>> A triset is made up of three exercises performed back to back with no rest. You can do a triset with just about any muscle group, although it works best with smaller body parts. For example, combining a move for the deltoid's front, middle, and rear heads effectively works the muscle from all major angles.

>> A giant set consists of four or more exercises done back to back. Think of it as a kind of circuit training in which you work one muscle group during the entire circuit of sets, moving quickly from one exercise to another and keeping your heart rate relatively high. Giant sets are typically done with larger, complex muscle groups, such as back, chest, and legs.

## GUIDE TO SUPERSETS

Supersets consist of two exercises for opposing muscle groups or a single body part performed back to back with no rest in between. When training antagonist muscle groups such as biceps and triceps, you'll be slightly stronger than usual on the second move, but when doing two exercises for the same muscle group, you'll be more fatigued and weaker than usual on the second exercise. Rest only after you complete both exercises, and repeat for the suggested number of sets.

>> The arms superset uses the same weighted EZ-bar for both moves. Because it works opposing muscle groups, you may be able to go fairly heavy.

>> Two is about the max number of machines you can expect to lay claim to at any given time at the gym without aggravating other gym members. This machine superset for legs starts off with a multijoint move and finishes with a single-joint one, allowing you to push those muscle fibers in your quads to the limit without having to worry about balancing the weight.

### ARMS SUPERSET (FOR ANTAGONIST MUSCLES) *

| EXERCISE | SETS | REPS |
| --- | --- | --- |
| Standing EZ-Bar Curl | 3 | 8-10 |
| Lying Triceps Extension | 3 | 8-10 |

*The next time you train arms with supersets, do the triceps move first.*

### LEGS SUPERSET

| EXERCISE | SETS | REPS |
| --- | --- | --- |
| Leg Press | 3 | 8-10 |
| Leg Extension | 3 | 8-10 |

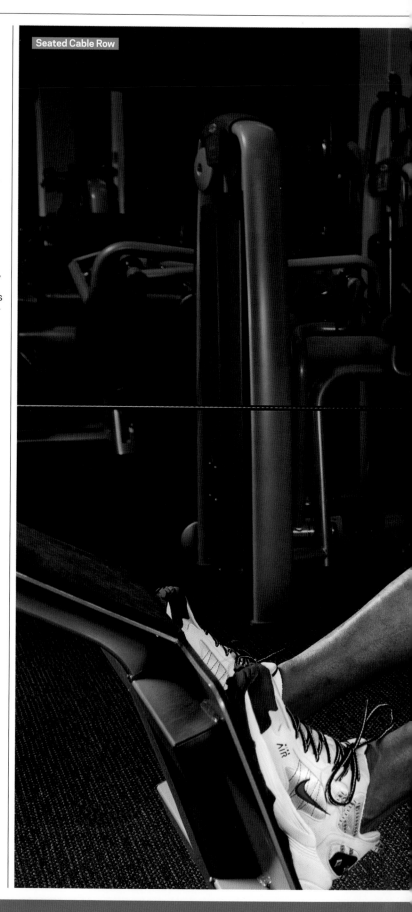

Seated Cable Row

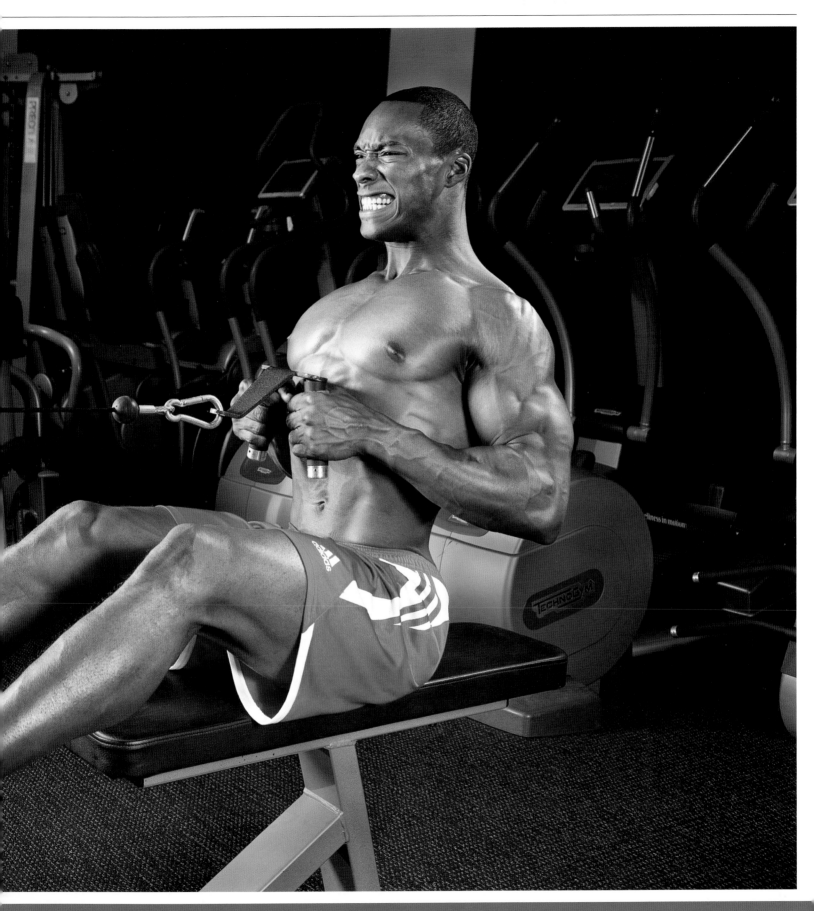

# INFUSING YOUR ROUTINE

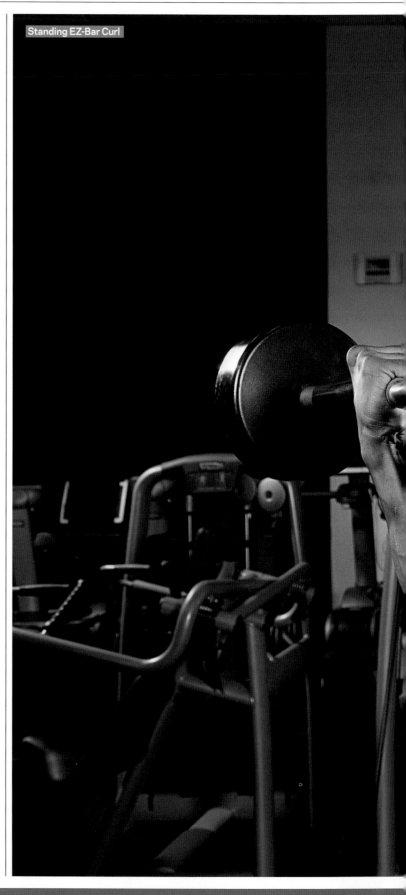

Standing EZ-Bar Curl

These techniques aren't recommended for beginners, who should be more concerned with proper technique and building a solid foundation, which can best be accomplished by straight-sets training. Using sets of multiple exercises is best for intermediate- to advanced-level lifters who want to kick-start a workout, get ripped, or just get in and out of the gym quickly.

>> Whether you combine two, three, or four exercises, start with the most demanding move, typically a compound (multijoint) move like the squat, then follow up with successively easier moves, including single-joint exercises. "While there are no hard-and-fast rules for using these methods, it may be better to use a compound movement first," Scheett says. "Isolation exercises are an ideal way to finish off a triset or a giant set, as they allow you to completely focus on the muscle group you're training."

>> Choose exercises that work the muscle somewhat differently. For example, start a chest superset with a flat-bench dumbbell press followed by a flye movement, or begin with the incline barbell press followed by decline flyes. Include moves in your sequence that will work the target muscle from different angles. If you choose exercises that target a similar area of the muscle group, begin with the free-weight version, then use a machine on the last set (such as dumbbell shoulder press to machine shoulder press).

>> Don't go too heavy. Linking several exercises for a single muscle group makes for one set of perhaps 20–30 reps, so choose your weights wisely. Go too heavy and you'll invite bad form and risk injury. Instead, select a lighter weight and go for reps; you'll more than make up for the weight with intensity.

>> Use a moderate rep speed. Even though you'll use a relatively lighter weight for higher total reps, do each rep deliberately and with full focus to get the most out of it.

>> Take a longer rest after the sequence is completed. Since you're more fatigued than if you'd done straight sets, take a slightly longer rest period after each circuit—as much as four minutes if you're doing giant sets, says Scheett—or about as much time as it takes you to catch your breath.

>> Don't overuse. If used too often, this high-intensity technique can contribute to overtraining and halt muscle growth. "Use supersets, trisets, and giant sets sparingly and for short periods," Scheett says.

>> If you want to get bigger and leaner, do superset training toward the end of your workout. Begin your routine with mass- and strength-building sets in the lower rep ranges with straight sets and plenty of rest, then finish off with supersets, trisets, or giant sets to get the best of both worlds.

>> Safely cheat. Keep your compound moves strict, but when fatigue really sets in, a little momentum can get you over the hump. Let your experience guide you as to how much cheating is safe, and enlist a spotter if possible.

>> Do machines last. Generally, free-weight exercises are more demanding than machine moves, so when linking the two, do the machine move last because you don't need to worry about balancing the weight.

>> Don't be a machine hog. Trying to monopolize three to four pieces of gym equipment at once is unreasonable, especially for people who are trying to work in. Unless it's very slow at your club, combine several exercises that you can do at a single station.

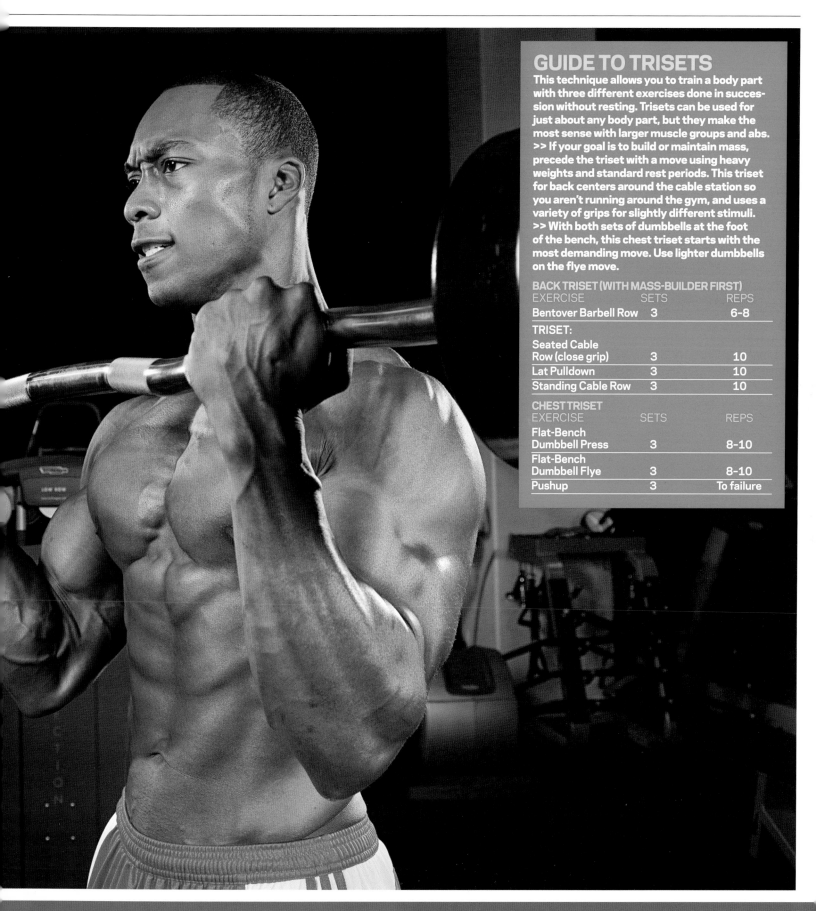

## GUIDE TO TRISETS

This technique allows you to train a body part with three different exercises done in succession without resting. Trisets can be used for just about any body part, but they make the most sense with larger muscle groups and abs. >> If your goal is to build or maintain mass, precede the triset with a move using heavy weights and standard rest periods. This triset for back centers around the cable station so you aren't running around the gym, and uses a variety of grips for slightly different stimuli. >> With both sets of dumbbells at the foot of the bench, this chest triset starts with the most demanding move. Use lighter dumbbells on the flye move.

### BACK TRISET (WITH MASS-BUILDER FIRST)

| EXERCISE | SETS | REPS |
| --- | --- | --- |
| Bentover Barbell Row | 3 | 6-8 |
| TRISET: | | |
| Seated Cable Row (close grip) | 3 | 10 |
| Lat Pulldown | 3 | 10 |
| Standing Cable Row | 3 | 10 |

### CHEST TRISET

| EXERCISE | SETS | REPS |
| --- | --- | --- |
| Flat-Bench Dumbbell Press | 3 | 8-10 |
| Flat-Bench Dumbbell Flye | 3 | 8-10 |
| Pushup | 3 | To failure |

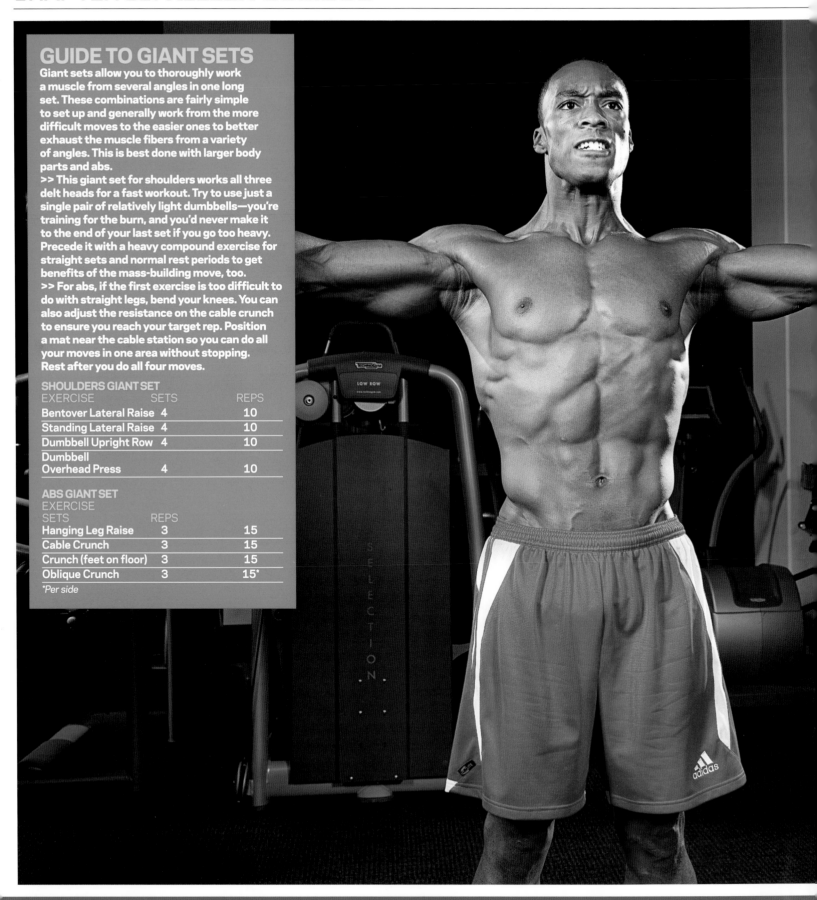

## GUIDE TO GIANT SETS

Giant sets allow you to thoroughly work a muscle from several angles in one long set. These combinations are fairly simple to set up and generally work from the more difficult moves to the easier ones to better exhaust the muscle fibers from a variety of angles. This is best done with larger body parts and abs.

>> This giant set for shoulders works all three delt heads for a fast workout. Try to use just a single pair of relatively light dumbbells—you're training for the burn, and you'd never make it to the end of your last set if you go too heavy. Precede it with a heavy compound exercise for straight sets and normal rest periods to get benefits of the mass-building move, too.

>> For abs, if the first exercise is too difficult to do with straight legs, bend your knees. You can also adjust the resistance on the cable crunch to ensure you reach your target rep. Position a mat near the cable station so you can do all your moves in one area without stopping. Rest after you do all four moves.

### SHOULDERS GIANT SET

| EXERCISE | SETS | REPS |
|---|---|---|
| Bentover Lateral Raise | 4 | 10 |
| Standing Lateral Raise | 4 | 10 |
| Dumbbell Upright Row | 4 | 10 |
| Dumbbell Overhead Press | 4 | 10 |

### ABS GIANT SET

| EXERCISE | SETS | REPS |
|---|---|---|
| Hanging Leg Raise | 3 | 15 |
| Cable Crunch | 3 | 15 |
| Crunch (feet on floor) | 3 | 15 |
| Oblique Crunch | 3 | 15* |

*Per side

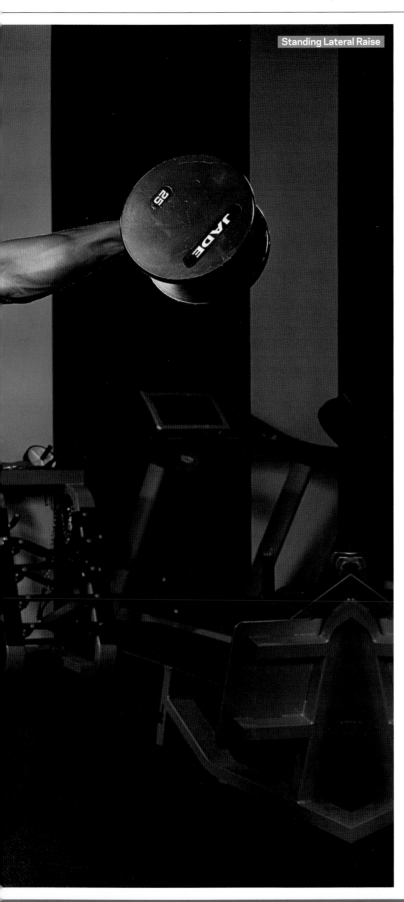

Standing Lateral Raise

# COMBO BENEFITS

>> More work in less time. Performing exercises back to back cuts your workout time without necessarily reducing the number of sets you perform since you spend less time resting.

>> Greater intensity. "Using multiple exercises to train the same muscle group without any rest between sets increases the intensity and places greater demands on the muscle fibers being trained," says Tim Scheett, Ph.D., assistant professor of exercise science at the College of Charleston (South Carolina). "This also increases the growth-hormone response during and following the workout, which will help increase muscle mass and decrease body fat."

>> Burn more body fat. Continuous work keeps your heart rate high, speeding your metabolism and burning more calories, which helps increase fat loss. "Due to the large volume and high intensity associated with giant sets, this method is ideal for contest preparation, aiding in muscle definition, and muscular detail by burning more calories within a given training session," Scheett adds.

>> Adds variety to your workout. This not only reduces boredom but helps you overcome plateaus by forcing you to train outside of your comfort zone or by shocking a lagging muscle group. "For intermediate or advanced trainees, these techniques offer an alternative method to gaining mass, particularly if you've reached a plateau in your training," explains Michael McGuigan, Ph.D., lecturer in exercise physiology at Edith Cowan University in Perth, Western Australia. "Supersets, trisets, and giant sets stimulate the muscles differently, and when a new stimulus is used, the muscle is forced to respond."

>> Get bigger and stronger. "These methods allow large amounts of volume to be performed in a short period," Scheett says. "Research has shown that performing high volumes of resistance exercise with very short rest periods between sets is very effective at increasing muscle size. This is due to the surge in lactate that's produced and the resulting rise in the amount of growth hormone being released. Research also shows increases in the amount of testosterone and other growth factors that are released with resistance training using high-intensity methods and very short rest periods between exercises."

"By incorporating supersets for opposing muscle groups specifically, you can also expect to get stronger," McGuigan adds. "Research from Australia using professional rugby players has shown that a muscle will be stronger if it's preceded by the contraction of its opposing muscle group, or antagonist. This is because when you train with straight sets, the muscle you're training is somewhat limited by its antagonist. For example, when training biceps with curls, the triceps muscle will inhibit contraction of the biceps to some extent. By performing a superset using dumbbell curls and triceps extensions, you'll be stronger on the triceps extension [the second exercise in the pairing]. For this reason, supersets are a very good method for increasing strength and muscle size."

>> Improve muscle recovery. "When performing a superset with leg curls and leg extensions, for example, the contraction of the quads during leg extensions boosts blood flow to the hamstrings (and vice versa) and could potentially aid in recovery by providing more nutrients and hormones to the muscle and also by removing waste products," McGuigan notes.

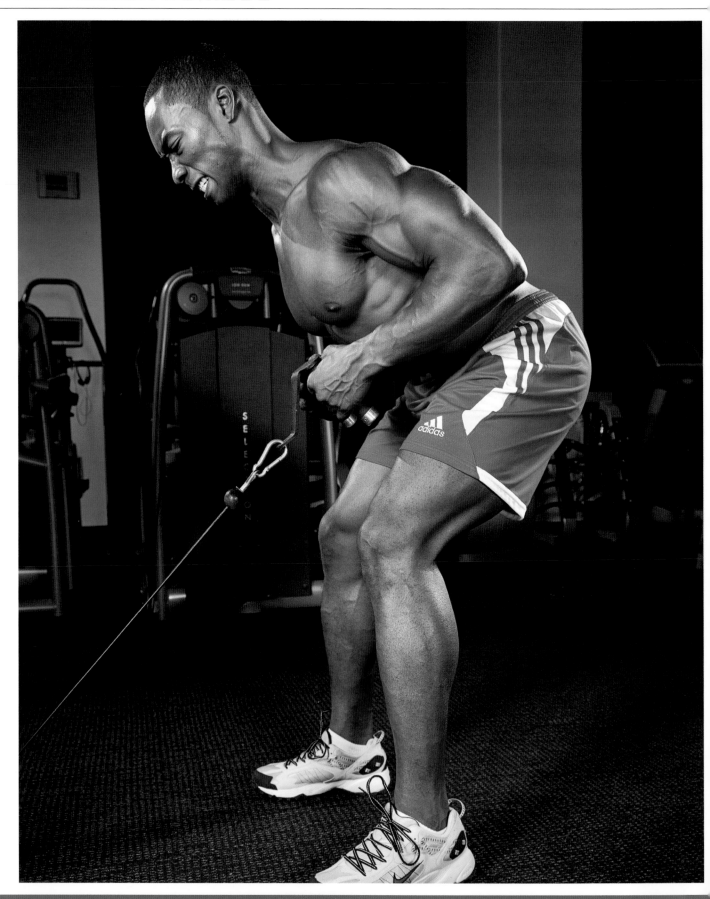

Standing
Cable Row

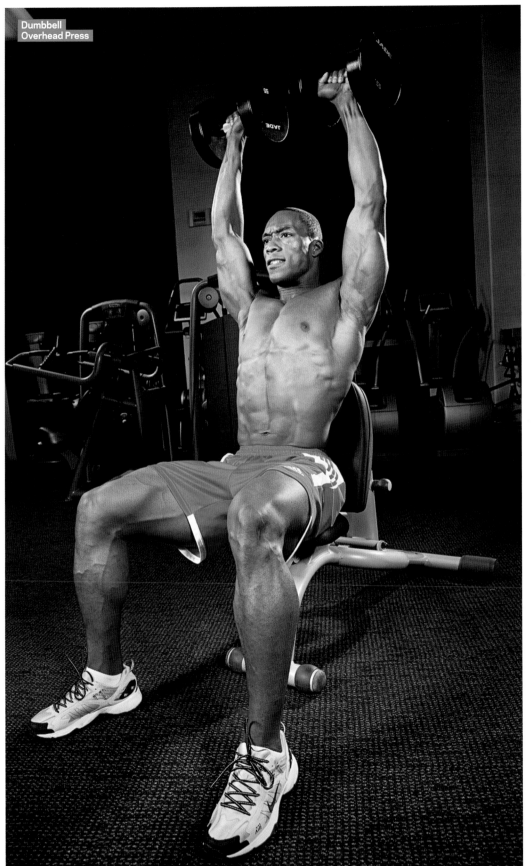

**Dumbbell Overhead Press**

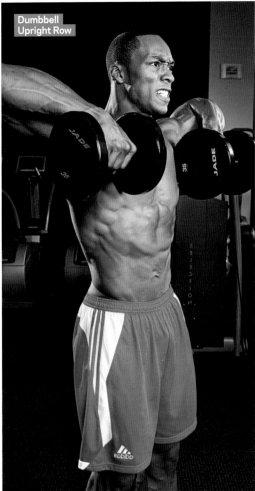

**Dumbbell Upright Row**

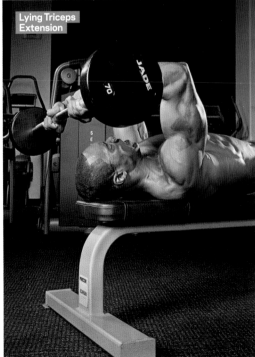

**Lying Triceps Extension**

# 50
# RULES OF
# FAT BURNING

*Muscle & Fitness* collects the strongest clinical research from around the world, bringing you dozens of tips to melt the flab from your abs.

**W**hatever you're doing isn't working to your satisaction. Why else would you be reading this? You swapped fried chicken for grilled and your treadmill is finally getting more attention than your TiVo. But your body isn't quite where you want it to be. Don't worry: Your bag of fat-burning tricks isn't empty yet. We've collected 50 comprehensive tips, all backed by more science than a NASA shuttle launch. By the time you've incorporated these fat-burning gems, we'll have 50 more for you. But by then, you probably won't need them.

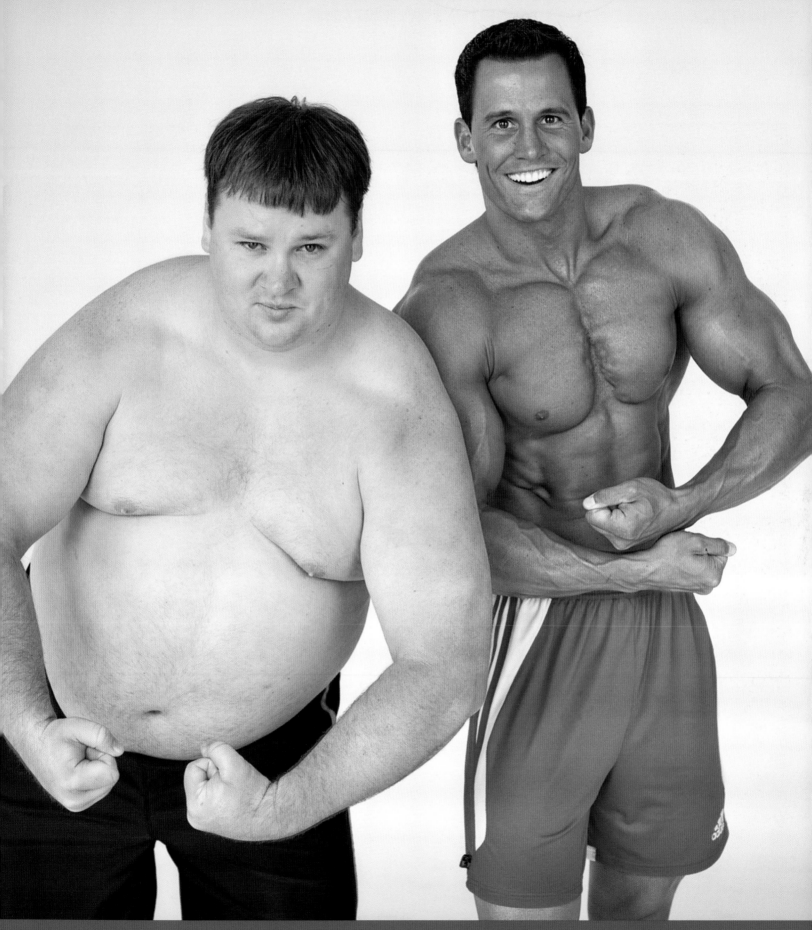

# WHAT YOU EAT

Getting lean obviously relies heavily on a solid nutrition plan. So it should come as no surprise that what and how you eat can have a big impact on your success. Use these 11 food rules to amp up your fat-burning potential.

## 1. GO PRO

A high-protein diet not only promotes hypertrophy but also enhances fat loss. Researchers at Skidmore College (Saratoga Springs, NY) found that when subjects followed a high-protein diet—40% of total daily calories from protein—for eight weeks, they lost significantly more body fat, particularly abdominal fat, than those following a low-fat/high-carb diet. One reason eating more protein may work is that it boosts levels of peptide YY, a hormone produced by gut cells that travels to the brain to decrease hunger and increase satiety.

## 2. SLOW DOWN

When you reach for carbs, choose slow-digesting whole grains such as brown rice, oatmeal, and whole-wheat bread, which keep insulin levels low and steady and prevent insulin spikes from halting fat burning and ramping up fat storing. A study conducted by researchers at Pennsylvania State University found that subjects following a low-calorie diet with carbs coming only from whole grains lost significantly more abdominal fat than those following a low-calorie diet with carbs from refined sources.

## 3. GET FAT

Not only will certain fats—particularly omega-3s—not lead to fat gain, but they can actually promote fat loss. Eating fat to lose fat seems counterintuitive, but if you keep your fat intake at about 30% of your total daily calories by choosing fatty fish such as salmon, sardines, or trout as well as other healthy fat sources such as olive oil, peanut butter, and walnuts, you can actually boost your fat loss compared to eating a low-fat diet.

## 4. EGG YOU ON

Eggs are packed with protein and have been shown to promote muscle strength and mass, and research shows that subjects consuming eggs for breakfast not only eat fewer calories throughout the day but also lose significantly more body fat. We recommend eating eggs for breakfast daily, scrambling three whole eggs with three egg whites.

## 5. UNFORBIDDEN FRUIT

A study from the Scripps Clinic in San Diego reported that subjects eating half a grapefruit or drinking eight ounces of grapefruit juice three times a day while otherwise eating normally lost an average of four pounds in 12 weeks, with some test subjects losing more than 10 pounds without dieting. The researchers suggest the effect is likely due to grapefruit's ability to reduce insulin levels. Try adding half a grapefruit to a few of your meals such as breakfast, lunch, and pre-workout.

## 6. MILK IT

Dairy products are rich in calcium, which can help spur fat loss, particularly around your abs. This may be due to the fact that calcium regulates the hormone calcitriol, which causes the body to produce fat and inhibit fat burning. When calcium levels are adequate, calcitriol and fat production are suppressed while fat burning is enhanced. Adding low-fat versions of cottage cheese and yogurt (Greek or plain) to your diet are great ways to boost protein intake and aid fat loss.

## 7. AN APPLE A DAY

Apples are a great slow-digesting carb that contain numerous beneficial antioxidants. One group of compounds known as apple polyphenols has been found to boost muscle strength, endurance, and even fat loss, especially from around the abs. While apple polyphenols appear to directly decrease body fat by increasing the activity of genes that enhance fat burning and decrease fat production and storage, the boost in endurance and strength can help further fat loss by allowing you to train harder longer. A typical large apple provides about 200 milligrams of apple polyphenols and about 30 grams of carbs.

## 8. SPICE IT UP

Hot peppers contain the active ingredient capsaicin, a chemical that has been shown to promote calorie burning at rest as well as reduce hunger and food intake. Its effects are particularly enhanced when used with caffeine, and research also shows that it boosts fat-burning during exercise. Try adding crushed red pepper, hot peppers, or hot pepper sauce to your meals to burn extra calories and fat. If you can't stand the heat, try supplements that contain capsaicin.

## 9. GO NUTS

A study from Loma Linda University in California reported that subjects following a low-calorie, higher-fat diet (40% of total calories from fat), with the majority of fat coming from almonds, lost significantly more body fat and fat around the abs in 24 weeks than subjects consuming the same calories but more carbs and less fat. So be sure to include nuts such as almonds, Brazil nuts, macadamia nuts, and walnuts in your diet.

## 10. BE MULTI-ORGANIC

Sure, it's pricier, but organic beef and dairy are worth the extra bucks. U.K. scientists found that organic milk had about 70% more omega-3 fatty acids than conventional milk, and a study published in the *Journal of Dairy Science* found that grass-fed cows produced milk containing 500% more conjugated linoleic acid (CLA) than cows who ate grain. Meat from organically raised cattle also contains higher levels of CLA and omega-3 fats. Since omega-3s and CLA can help you drop fat as well as gain muscle, it makes sense to shell out the extra cash for organic cheese, cottage cheese, milk, and yogurt as well as grass-fed beef.

## 11. ADD SOME GUAC

Avocados are full of monounsaturated fat, which isn't generally stored as body fat. They also contain mannoheptulose, a sugar that actually blunts insulin release and enhances calcium absorption. As mentioned earlier, keeping insulin low at most times of day is critical for encouraging fat loss, and getting adequate calcium can also promote fat loss. Try adding a quarter of an avocado to salads and sandwiches.

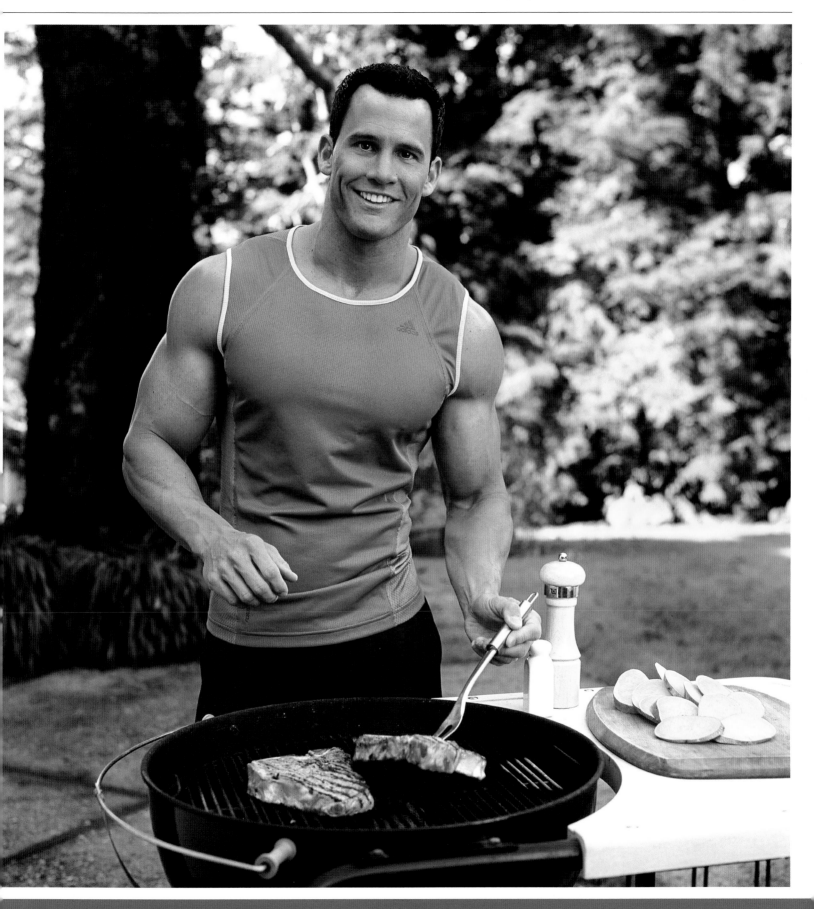

# WHAT YOU DRINK

Beverages can play an important role in your ability to drop fat. Consider sipping (or passing) on these eight beverages to get extra-lean.

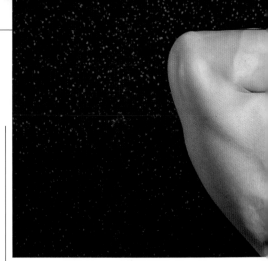

## 12. GO GREEN

The main ingredient in green tea, epigallocatechin gallate (EGCG), inhibits the enzyme that normally breaks down the neurohormone norepinephrine. Norepinephrine keeps the metabolic rate up, so preventing its breakdown helps you burn more calories throughout the day. Drinking green tea is a great way to stay hydrated during workouts, as a new study in the *Journal of Nutrition* reported that subjects drinking green tea and exercising lost significantly more abdominal fat than those drinking a placebo.

## 13. IN THE BLACK

Green, oolong, and black teas all come from the same plant, but different processing causes black and oolong teas to lose their green color and turn brownish/black. Oolong tea has been shown to enhance metabolic rate due to polyphenols other than EGCG. Black tea may also aid fat loss: Researchers from University College London reported that black tea consumption can help reduce levels of cortisol, which encourages fat storage especially around the midsection.

## 14. BE AQUA MAN

German researchers have shown that drinking about two cups of cold water can temporarily boost metabolic rate by roughly 30%. The effect appears to be mainly due to an increase in norepinephrine.

## 15. GET ENERGIZED

Certain energy drinks have been shown to boost fat loss. University of Oklahoma researchers reported in a 2008 study that when 60 male and female subjects consumed a diet energy drink containing 200mg of caffeine and 250mg of EGCG from green tea extract for 28 days, they lost more than one pound of body fat without changing their diets or exercise habits.

## 16. WHEY LEAN

Drinking whey protein as a between-meals snack is a smart way to enhance not only muscle growth but also fat loss. U.K. researchers found that when subjects consumed a whey protein shake 90 minutes before eating a buffet-style meal, they ate significantly less food than when they consumed a casein shake beforehand. The scientists reported that this was due to whey's ability to boost levels of the hunger-blunting hormones cholecystokinin and glucagonlike peptide-1.

## 17. SAY SOY-ANARA TO FAT

Soy protein is a proven fat burner. In fact, in a 2008 review paper, University of Alabama-Birmingham researchers concluded that soy protein can aid fat loss, possibly by decreasing appetite and calorie intake. The scientists also found that subjects drinking 20 grams of soy daily for three months lost a significant amount of abdominal fat.

## 18. GET THICK

When you whip up a protein shake, consider making it thicker by using less water. It could help you feel less hungry while dieting. In a study from Purdue University, subjects drank two shakes that were identical in nutritional content and reported significantly greater and more prolonged reductions in hunger after drinking the thicker shake.

## 19. NOT SO SWEET

Even though artificially sweetened drinks are calorie-free, drinking too many can actually hinder your fat-loss progress. It seems that beverages like diet soda mess with your brain's ability to regulate calorie intake, causing you to feel hungrier than normal so you eat more total calories. Other research suggests that the sweet taste of these drinks can increase the release of insulin, which can blunt fat burning and enhance fat storage.

# WHAT SUPPLEMENTS YOU TAKE

While whole foods are the key element to getting lean, supplements can provide a potent fat-burning stimulus. Consider using these six supps.

## 20. GO EVEN GREENER

The majority of studies showing the effectiveness of green tea for fat loss have used green tea extract. One study confirmed that the EGCG from the extract was absorbed significantly better than the EGCG from the tea. Take about 500mg of green tea extract in the morning and afternoon before meals.

## 21. SEE CLA

You'll also want to add the healthy fat CLA to your supplement regimen. CLA can significantly aid fat loss while simultaneously enhancing hypertrophy and strength gains. Research shows it can even help specifically target ab fat.

## 22. GO FISH

As mentioned in tip No. 3, the essential omega-3 fats in fish oil promote fat loss, which is enhanced with exercise. This is also true for fish-oil supplements containing omega-3 fats. Take 1–2g of fish oil at breakfast, lunch, and dinner.

## 23. YOU BET YOUR ASTAXANTHIN

Japanese researchers reported in a 2008 study that mice supplemented with astaxanthin, combined with an exercise program, for four weeks saw accelerated fat burning, greater fat loss, and enhanced endurance compared with mice that did just exercise. The scientists determined that astaxanthin protects the system that transports fat into the mitochondria of muscle cells, where it's burned as fuel. Take 4mg of astaxanthin with food once or twice per day, with one dose taken with your pre-workout meal.

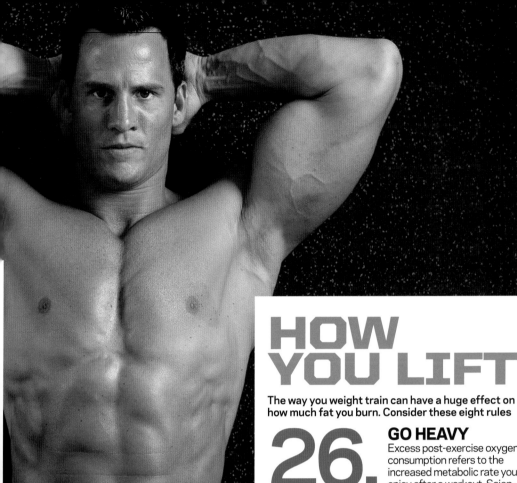

### 24. GO COMMERCIAL

A 2009 study reported that lifters taking the fat-burning supplement Meltdown by VPX (containing caffeine, synephrine, yohimbine, and beta-phenylethylamine, to name a few) burned 30% more calories and had a more than 40% increase in markers of lipolysis (fat release from fat cells) for the 90 minutes after working out compared to when subjects consumed a placebo. Regardless of the brand of thermogenic you choose, always follow label instructions and take the other five supplements mentioned here as well (starting at rule 20) to maximize fat-burning.

### 25. CARRY MORE FAT AWAY WITH CARNITINE

This amino acid–like compound is critical for carrying fat in the body to the mitochondria of cells, where it's burned away for good. Research confirms that taking carnitine when dieting can help maximize fat-burning efforts. Take 1–2g of carnitine in the form of L-carnitine, L-carnitine L-tartrate, or glycine propionyl-L-carnitine.

# HOW YOU LIFT

The way you weight train can have a huge effect on how much fat you burn. Consider these eight rules

### 26. GO HEAVY

Excess post-exercise oxygen consumption refers to the increased metabolic rate you enjoy after a workout. Scientists at the Norwegian University of Sport and Physical Education analyzed multiple studies and found that training with heavier weights for fewer reps produces a greater rise in resting metabolic rate that'll last longer compared with training with lighter weights and doing more reps. Although most guys may think they need to train with higher reps to burn more fat, you still want to lift heavy (3–7 reps) some of the time to maximize the calories and fat you burn when you're not at the gym.

### 27. GO LIGHT

While lifting heavy does burn more calories post-workout, performing higher reps burns more calories during the workout, as College of New Jersey researchers reported at a 2007 annual meeting of the National Strength and Conditioning Association. Be sure to mix up your training by using lighter weight and higher reps (10–20) during some workouts and heavy weight and low reps (3–7) in others. Another way to get the best of both worlds is to perform four sets of most exercises, doing your first two sets with heavy weight and low reps and the last two with light weight and high reps.

### 28. REST LESS

Researchers from the College of New Jersey also discovered that when subjects rested 30 seconds between sets on the bench press, they burned more than 50% more calories than when they rested three minutes. To maximize fat loss, keep your workout moving by resting less than a minute between sets.

### 29. FORCE IT

A study on collegiate football players found that using a high-intensity weight program—just one set per exercise for 6–10 reps to failure, plus forced reps and a static contraction for several seconds—caused more body fat loss in 10 weeks than a lower-intensity program consisting of three sets of 6–10 reps per exercise taken just to muscle failure. This could be due to a greater hike in growth hormone (GH) in the high-intensity group: In a study from Finland, forced reps boosted GH three times higher than training to failure. Go past failure when trying to get lean by using forced reps, static contractions, rest-pause, or dropsets.

### 30. BE FREE

Using free weights, especially in multijoint moves such as squats, has been found to burn more calories than doing similar exercises on machines like the leg press. Scientists said the difference may be due to the greater number of stabilizer muscles used during multijoint exercises done with free weights.

### 31. FEEL THE NEED FOR SPEED

Fast, explosive reps burn more calories than the typical slow, controlled reps you're used to doing in the gym, say researchers from Ball State University in Indiana. They believe that because fast-twitch muscle fibers are less energy-efficient than their slow-twitch counterparts, they burn more fuel during exercise. To perform fast reps in your workouts, choose a weight equal to 30–60% of your one-rep max (or a weight you can lift for 15–35 reps) for each exercise. Do your first two sets with 3–8 fast reps, then follow with 2–3 sets of normal-paced reps.

### 32. BE NEGATIVE

In one recent study, subjects who performed a negative-rep workout of three sets of bench presses and squats increased their GH levels by almost 4,000%. Since GH frees up fat from fat cells, using negative reps may help you shed extra body fat. To add negatives to your routine, either have a spotter help you get 3–5 negative reps after reaching failure on a regular set, or load the bar with about 120% of your one-rep max and have a spotter help you perform five negative reps that take you 3–5 seconds each to complete.

### 33. TUNE IN

Listening to your own music can boost your workout intensity and fat-loss efforts. A study conducted by the Weider Research Group and presented at the 2008 annual meeting of the National Strength and Conditioning Association found that trained subjects listening to their own music selection could complete significantly more reps than when they trained without their preferred music.

# HOW YOU RUN

**Cardio, obviously, is a primary component of getting lean. It's the easiest way to burn the most calories during exercise. Use these eight rules to help you maximize your fat loss.**

## 34. GO AFTER IT

Do your cardio after you hit the weights. Japanese researchers found that when subjects performed cardio after resistance training, they burned significantly more fat than when they did cardio first. The scientists also reported that fat burning was maximal during the first 15 minutes of cardio following the weight workout, so hit the stationary bike, elliptical machine, or treadmill after you lift, even if it's for just 15 minutes.

## 35. HIIT IT

The best way to burn the most fat with cardio is via high-intensity interval training (HIIT). This involves doing intervals of high-intensity exercise (such as running at 90% of your max heart rate) followed by intervals of low-intensity exercise (walking at a moderate pace) or rest. A litany of research confirms that this burns more fat than the continuous, steady-state cardio most people do at a moderate intensity, such as walking for 30 minutes at 60–70% of their max heart rates.

## 36. STAGGER IT

In one study, subjects who did three 10-minute bouts of running separated by 20-minute rest periods found the workout easier than when they ran at the same intensity for 30 minutes. The intermittent cardio even burned more fat and has also been shown to burn more calories post-workout than the same amount of continuous exercise.

## 37. FASHIONABLY LATE

The time of day you do your cardio can impact how many calories you burn post-workout. University of Wisconsin-La Crosse researchers reported that highly trained subjects who performed 30 minutes of stationary cycling between 5 p.m. and 7 p.m. raised their metabolic rates higher post-workout than when they did the same cardio exercise between 5 a.m. and 7 a.m. or between 11 a.m. and 1 p.m. While your best bet is to train whenever it best fits your schedule, try training in the evening to enhance your post-workout calorie burn.

## 38. BE SCOTTISH

University of Edinburgh (Scotland) researchers reported that when subjects did four to six 30-second sprints on a stationary cycle separated by four minutes of rest for just two weeks, their blood-glucose and insulin levels were reduced by almost 15% and 40%, respectively, and insulin sensitivity improved by about 25% following consumption of 75g of glucose. Keeping insulin levels low and steady can help maximize fat burning and minimize fat storage. So even if you don't have 20-30 minutes for a cardio workout, doing just 2-3 minutes of sprinting can at least help keep insulin down and fat burning up.

## 39. CLIMB IT

Consider other forms of cardio. A recent study from Italy found that when subjects rock-climbed, their average heart rates were about 80% of their max, which equates to a pretty intense cardio session. In addition, subjects burned about 12 calories per minute for a 180-pound guy, or just less than 400 calories in 30 minutes. Check out indoor or outdoor rock-climbing sites in your area.

## 40. KICK IT

Another way to get your cardio is with martial arts. Wayne State College (Nebraska) researchers found that when beginning martial artists performed a tae kwon do workout—cycling between front kicks, butterfly stretches, forearm strikes, crunches, side kicks, quad stretches, and pushups—their heart rates rose 80%, and they burned about 300 calories per half-hour. Besides tae kwon do, you can try aikido, jiu-jitsu, judo, karate, kung fu, or any other style of martial arts.

## 41. SPIT IT OUT

University of Birmingham (United Kingdom) scientists found that when trained cyclists rode as fast as possible while rinsing their mouths with a beverage similar to a sports drink and spitting it out every seven to eight minutes, they could cover a certain mileage three minutes faster than when they rinsed with water. We don't suggest you try this in an indoor cycling class, but rinsing your mouth every 10 minutes with a sports drink and spitting it out could help you train at a higher intensity—without the added calories.

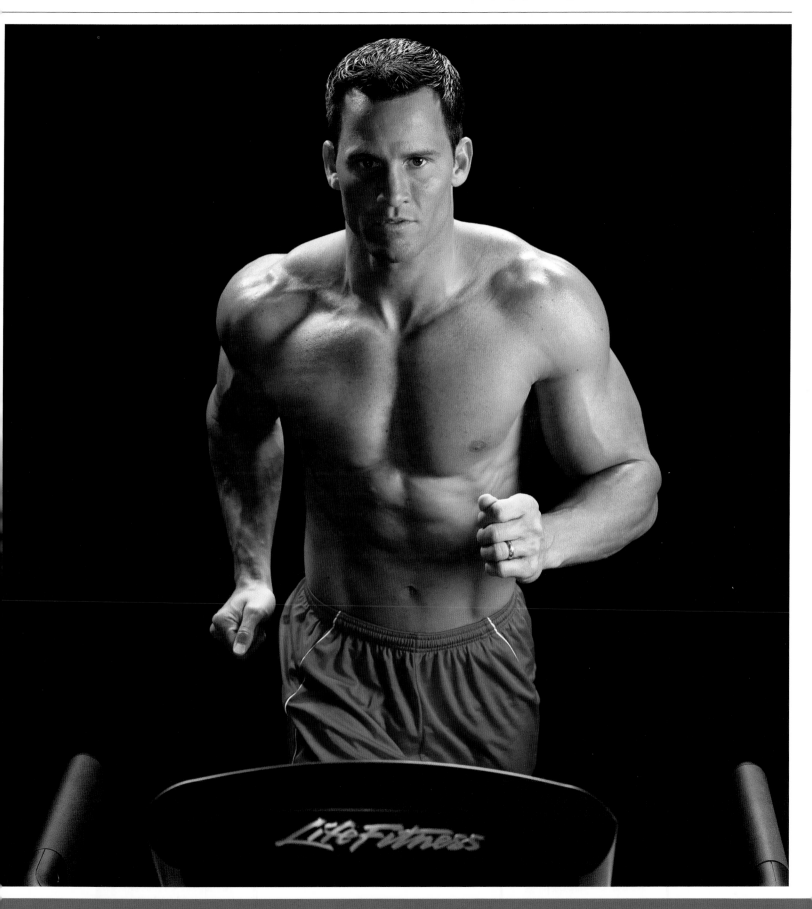

# OTHER RULES

Some things that can impact your ability to lose fat may not be directly related to what you eat or drink, or to your exercise routine. Still, these nine tips could aid fat loss.

## 42. GET UP

Research from Australia found that, out of 2,000-plus subjects who exercised vigorously for at least 2.5 hours per week, those who watched more than 40 minutes of television per day had higher waist circumferences than those watching less than 40 minutes. The scientists theorize that sitting for prolonged periods compromises the body's ability to burn fat, which was shown by University of Missouri–Columbia researchers in both animals and humans. Avoid this slump by getting up and stretching at least every 20 minutes while sitting at work or at home.

## 43. TAKE A PICTURE

A picture could be worth a thousand calories. Researchers from the University of Wisconsin-Madison found that test subjects who recorded with photographs what they ate for one week reported that the images triggered critical evaluation of the food before eating it, prompting them to make better food choices. This wasn't the case for subjects who simply wrote down what they ate. Try keeping a photo food log as well as a journal in which you calculate your macronutrient intake.

## 44. PORTION IT

One study from Cornell University reported that when moviegoers were given a large container (about 22 cups) of fresh popcorn during a movie, they ate 45% more than those given a medium container (about 11 cups). Even more disturbing was that subjects given a large container of stale popcorn still ate about 35% more than those given a medium container, even though they rated the popcorn's taste as bad. You can use this research in a couple of ways: For lean protein sources, give yourself a large amount; for side dishes such as rice, potatoes, and bread, keep the serving on the small side.

## 45. LAUGH IT OFF

Japanese scientists found that when subjects ate a 500-calorie meal while watching a 40-minute comedy show, their blood-glucose levels were much lower than when they consumed the same meal during a boring 40-minute lecture. The researchers suggest that laughter may have altered subjects' brain chemistry in such a way that glucose entered the blood more slowly, or blood glucose was taken up by the muscles more rapidly. Try eating meals while watching something funny on TV to keep your blood-glucose and insulin levels low to help encourage fat loss.

## 46. SLEEP ON IT

One study in the *American Journal of Epidemiology* reported that subjects sleeping five hours or less per night were one-third more likely to gain 30-plus pounds over the 16-year study than those who slept seven hours or longer per night. This may be due to an imbalance in the hormones leptin and ghrelin: While leptin decreases hunger and increases the metabolic rate, ghrelin boosts hunger. A study by University of Chicago researchers found that men who were sleep-deprived for two days experienced a rise in ghrelin levels and a drop in leptin levels, along with a concomitant rise in hunger. A Stanford University study showed that subjects who slept the least had lower levels of leptin and higher levels of ghrelin and body fat compared with those who slept eight hours. Try to get seven to nine hours of sleep every night to not only enhance your recovery but also aid your health and help keep fat off.

## 47. CHEW IT

A study done at Glasgow Caledonian University found that subjects who chewed gum between meals ate significantly less food at the second meal than those who didn't chew gum. The researchers concluded that chewing gum increases satiety and therefore reduces food intake.

## 48. BE A TRANSPORTER

Remember, any activity you do burns calories, and burning more calories than you consume is the most critical aspect of getting lean. So consider how far away certain destinations are such as work, the gym, the grocery store, and your friends' homes. Depending on the distance and the time you have, walk, or bike to burn more calories and fat.

## 49. FEEL THE VIBE

In a study from Stony Brook University, mice placed on a vibrating platform for 15 minutes a day for up to 15 weeks were found to have less body fat than mice not exposed to vibration. Research in humans has seen similar results with vibration exposure enhancing fat loss. If your gym has a vibration machine—often called a Power Plate—get a trainer to walk you through it and consider using it for a few minutes a couple of times per week.

## 50. BE A GAMER

The popular and very active video game *Dance Dance Revolution* can provide a great workout, according to researchers from the University of Wisconsin-La Crosse. They reported that adult subjects burned as many as 10 calories per minute playing the game, which is equivalent to a good run.

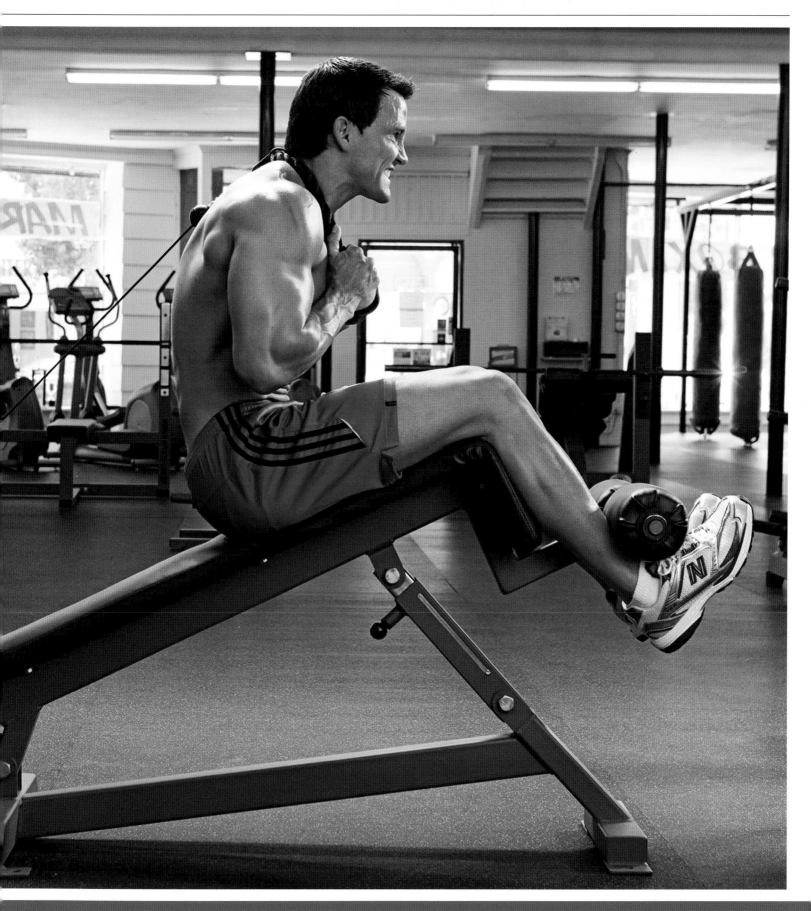

# CHAPTER 15

# FIT WITH HIIT

**Science has dropped the hammer on endless bouts of steady-state cardio. If you're looking to get totally peeled without burning through muscle mass, shorter durations are the answer.**

Less is more…except when it applies to things you really don't enjoy, that is. Take cardio, for example. How much cardio does it take to burn through that stubborn layer of fat lingering around your abdomen? Copious amounts—or at least that's what it feels like at times, since the most pervasive methodology behind fat burning involves seemingly interminable sessions of cardiovascular activity done at a sustained rate. Where cardio is concerned, the theory has always been more is more.

But all that's about to change. What would you say if we told you that the latest scientific research suggests shorter cardio sessions for crazy fat loss? How would you feel if you could actually end up burning more fat in the long run while holding on to more of your iron-wrought muscle? You can go ahead and smile—because it's entirely true. High-intensity interval training, or HIIT, is on the fast track to becoming the standard for steady and sustained fat loss.

With HIIT, the workouts are shorter, yes, but you'll actually be working harder than the guy on the treadmill next to you. HIIT is what it says—high-intensity—and the results are undeniable. If you're used to wearing a heart-rate monitor to judge the efficiency of your cardio, shelve it—you won't need it. By cycling between bouts of all-out effort and short stretches of active recovery, a mirror will be all you need to gauge your progress.

## BURNING DEBATE

Bodybuilders and others have long used steady-state cardio, which involves low- to moderate-intensity exercise performed at 60–70% of one's maximum heart rate (MHR), to whittle away body fat. Trainers and other experts argue that since lower-intensity cardio exercise burns a higher percentage of fat for energy, slow and steady indeed wins the race.

HIIT cardio, on the other hand, involves intervals of high-intensity exercise—at a rate near 90% MHR—followed by intervals of slower-paced active recovery. Anecdotal reports and early research on HIIT went against the steady-state establishment, claiming that it was the superior method of cardio for losing fat. And the exercise community, likely looking for a way to collectively limit its time on a conveyor belt, felt it was time for in-depth science to put an end to the developing debate. What they found, time after time, was that HIIT cardio was the best way to lose fat, despite the fact that it required less total time.

One of the earliest studies, done by researchers at Laval University in Quebec, Canada, kept it basic, using two groups in a months-long experiment. One group followed a 15-week program using HIIT while the other performed only steady-state cardio for 20 weeks. Proponents of steady-state training were pleased to hear that those subjects burned 15,000 calories more than their HIIT counterparts. Those who followed the HIIT program, however, lost significantly more body fat.

Another study from East Tennessee State University demonstrated similar findings with subjects who followed an eight-week HIIT program. Again, HIIT proved to be the better fat-burner—subjects dropped 2% body fat over the course of the experiment. Meanwhile, those who plodded through the eight weeks on a steady-state program lost no body fat.

The most recent study, out of Australia, reported that a group of females who followed a 20-minute HIIT program consisting of eight-second sprints followed by 12 seconds of rest lost an amazing six times more body fat than a group that followed a 40-minute cardio program performed at a constant intensity of 60% MHR.

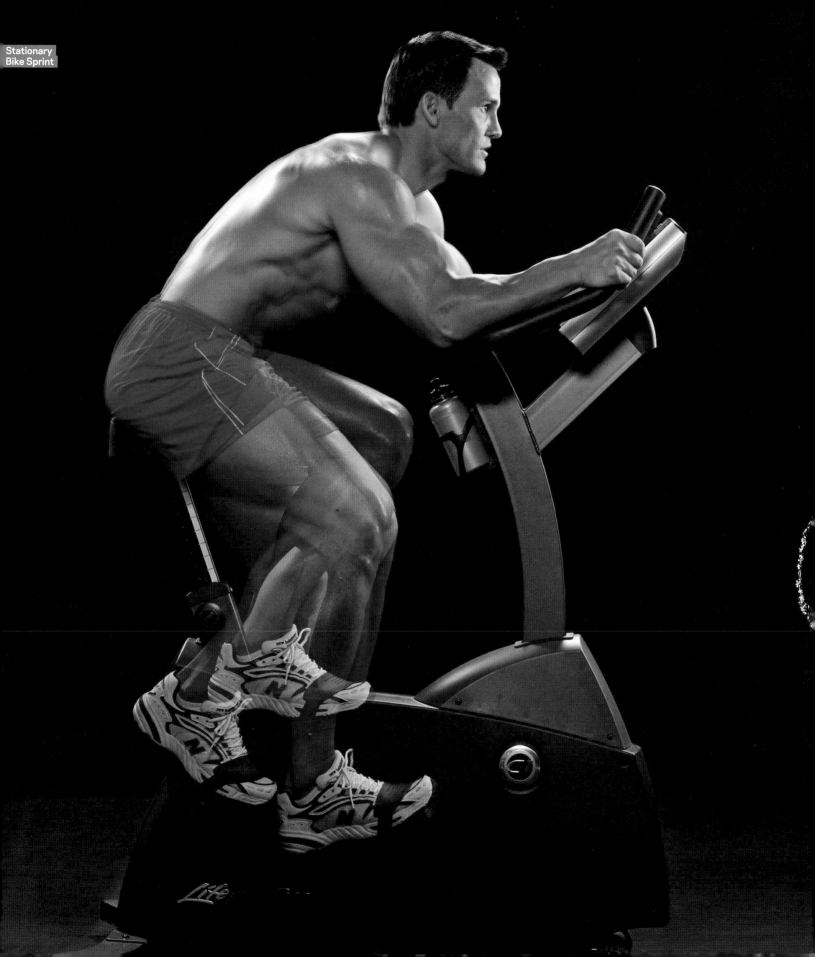

# TURN UP

So what is it about HIIT cardio training that sends body fat to the great beyond? There are actually several reasons, but the first and perhaps most important involves its effect on your metabolism.

A study from Baylor College of Medicine Iin Houston reported that subjects who performed a HIIT workout on a stationary cycle burned significantly more calories during the 24 hours following the workout than those who cycled at a moderate, steady-state intensity due to a rise in resting metabolism. Why? Since HIIT is tougher on the body, it requires more energy (read: calories) to repair itself afterward.

The previously mentioned East Tennessee State study found that test subjects in the HIIT program also burned nearly 100 more calories per day during the 24 hours after exercise. More recently, a study presented by Florida State University-Tallahassee researchers at the 2007 Annual Meeting of the American College of Sports Medicine (ACSM) reported that subjects who performed HIIT cardio burned almost 10% more calories during the 24 hours following exercise than a steady-state group, despite the fact that the total calories burned during each workout were the same.

Research also confirms that HIIT enhances the metabolic machinery in muscle cells that promotes fat burning and blunts fat production. The Laval University study discovered that the HIIT subjects' muscle fibers had significantly higher markers for fat oxidation (fat burning) than those in the steady-state exercise group. And a study published in a 2007 issue of the *Journal of Applied Physiology* reported that young females who performed seven HIIT workouts

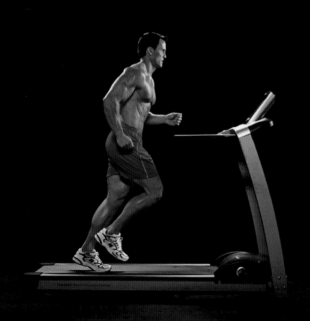 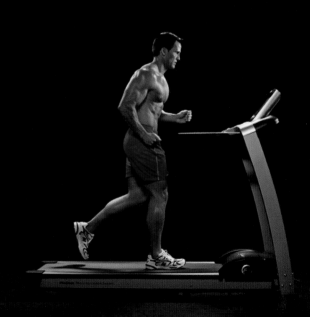

# THE HIIT

over a two-week period experienced a 30% increase in both fat oxidation and levels of muscle enzymes that enhance fat oxidation.

Moreover, researchers from the Norwegian University of Science and Technology reported that subjects with metabolic syndrome—a combination of medical disorders that increases one's risk of cardiovascular disease and diabetes—who followed a 16-week HIIT program had a 100% greater decrease in the fat-producing enzyme fatty acid synthase compared with subjects who followed a program of continuous moderate-intensity exercise.

The bonus to all this research is discovering that shorter exercise sessions will allow you to hold on to more muscle. Pro physique competitors often have to walk a fine line between just enough and too much steady-state cardio because the usual prescription of 45–60 minutes, sometimes done twice a day pre-contest, can rob muscles of size and fullness. Short, hard bursts of cardio, on the other hand, will help you preserve your hard-earned muscle mass.

To illustrate the point, think about the size of a marathon runner's legs compared to a sprinter's legs—the sprinter, whose entire training schedule revolves around HIIT, possesses significantly more muscular thighs. In the event you choose cycling as your primary method of HIIT cardio, you can actually add leg mass because of the increased recruitment of the growth-crazy, fast-twitch fibers in your thighs.

HIIT could be the only way to train for people looking to lose fat while adding and/or preserving muscle mass.

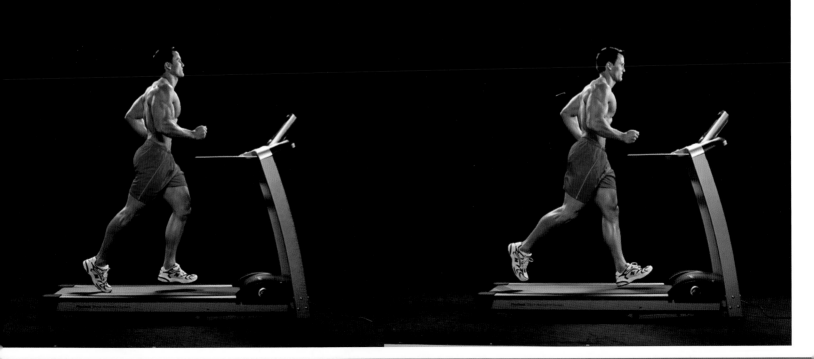

# REV IT UP

No one enjoys doing cardio, but it's a necessary component of reaching your fitness and physique goals. But that doesn't mean it needs to be monotonous to be effective, and we've shown you the science to prove it. Turning up the heat on your workouts with HIIT will keep your gym time feeling productive while speeding up your fat oxidation—and in less time than you'd normally spend doing cardio. If steady-state is the four-door sedan of cardio, HIIT is the Porsche—it's sexier, and there's enough under the hood to keep you blowing past the guy next to you.

## MAXIMIZING FAT BURNING

**Now that you know which cardio method works best for maximum fat loss, combine these tips with your HIIT cardio to speed your progress**

>> **Time your HIIT sessions.** Doing cardio after weights or in the morning on an empty stomach will burn the greatest amount of fat. During both of these times your body is slightly carb-depleted, making fat the primary fuel source for energy.

>> **Preserve muscle.** If you do cardio first thing in the morning, have a half-scoop of whey protein (about 10 grams) mixed in water or 6-10 grams of mixed amino acids pre-workout. This will help ensure your body draws most of its energy from fat and these fast-digesting supplements instead of your muscle.

>> **Make it an uphill climb.** Consider working hills into your HIIT cardio to add more detail to your hams and glutes. If you don't have hills available, adjust the incline on a treadmill to simulate it. Be sure to drop the incline to level, or zero, during low-intensity intervals.

>> **Get in and out.** Limit HIIT cardio sessions to 20-30 minutes to maximize intensity while actually aiding muscle growth and preventing muscle loss.

>> **Adjust for the lag.** During intervals on a treadmill, there will be a slight lag time as the machine adjusts to the change in speed: By the time the treadmill is up to running speed, the fast interval portion is almost over. To keep your intensity high, begin the sprint portion of the interval when the machine has reached your target speed. You can do this by counting seconds once the target speed is reached or by straddling the sides of the treadmill as it gets up to speed.

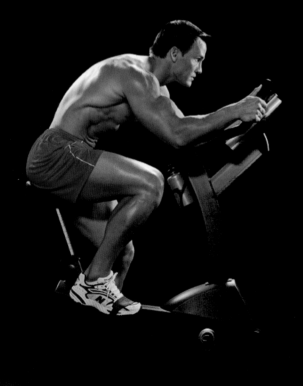
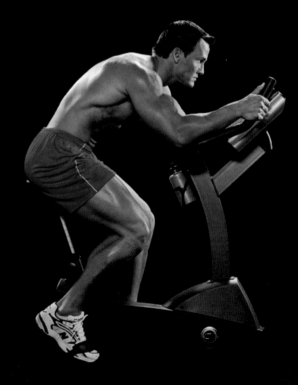

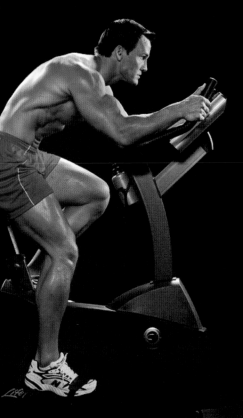

# MAKING HIIT WORK FOR YOU

Below are three sample HIIT cardio workouts. The training modes listed here are merely examples; feel free to substitute other cardio choices. The mode of training isn't as important as the method you use. Each sprint, whether on foot or a stationary cycle, indicates an all-out effort. The active-recovery intervals should be slow enough to get you ready for the next sprint. Start using these workouts to fine-tune your fat-fighting machine.

## TREADMILL SPRINT

| INTENSITY | TIME | INCLINE |
|---|---|---|
| Warmup | 2-3 min. | 0 |
| Walk | 1 min. | 0 |
| Sprint | 1 min. | 1 |
| Walk | 1 min. | 0 |
| Sprint | 1 min. | 1 |
| Walk | 1 min. | 0 |
| Sprint | 1 min. | 1 |
| Walk | 1 min. | 0 |
| Sprint | 1 min. | 3 |
| Walk | 1 min. | 0 |
| Sprint | 1 min. | 5 |
| Walk | 1 min. | 0 |
| Sprint | 1 min. | 5 |
| Walk | 1 min. | 0 |
| Sprint | 1 min. | 5 |
| Walk | 1 min. | 0 |
| Sprint | 1 min. | 5 |
| Walk | 1 min. | 0 |
| Sprint | 1 min. | 5 |
| Walk | 1 min. | 0 |
| Sprint | 1 min. | 5 |
| Walk | 1 min. | 0 |
| Sprint | 1 min. | 5 |
| Walk | 1 min. | 0 |
| Sprint | 1 min. | 5 |
| Cooldown | 2-3 min. | 0 |

Total: 28-30 min.

## OUTDOOR SPRINT

| INTENSITY | TIME |
|---|---|
| Warmup | 2-3 min. |
| Sprint | 10 sec. |
| Slow walk | 20 sec. |
| Sprint | 10 sec. |
| Slow walk | 20 sec. |
| Sprint | 10 sec. |
| Slow walk | 20 sec. |
| Sprint | 10 sec. |
| Slow walk | 20 sec. |

Perform circuit seven times for 14 minutes total.

### SLOW WALK

| | |
|---|---|
| Cooldown | 2-3 min. |

Total: 18-20 min.

*TIP: Consider the time it takes the treadmill to reach your incline and sprint speed by adjusting 5-10 seconds early.

## STATIONARY BIKE

| INTENSITY | TIME |
|---|---|
| Warmup | 2-3 min. |
| Sprint | 30 sec. |
| Slow pedal | 30 sec. |
| Sprint | 30 sec. |
| Slow pedal | 30 sec. |
| Sprint | 30 sec. |
| Slow pedal | 30 sec. |

Perform circuit eight times for 24 minutes total.

| | |
|---|---|
| Cooldown | 2-3 min. |

Total: 28-30 min.

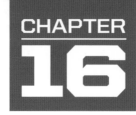

# CHAPTER 16

# FULL-METAL CARDIO

**Forgo mundane cardio workouts with this weightlifting circuit program and burn more fat in the process.**

It has to be some sort of proven training fact: You're not going to work as hard and make as much progress on exercises you despise versus those you enjoy doing. Case in point: When's the last time an elliptical session made you practically (or actually) puke in the trash can at the gym? Now think back to the last hardcore leg day you struggled through. Our guess is that the squats, heavy lunges, and step-ups were much more intense—and nauseating—than the cardio workout that allowed you to catch up on yesterday's *SportsCenter* highlights. And it's pretty much guaranteed that the intense lifting routine burned more total calories and body fat (during the workout and afterward combined) than the ESPN-sponsored one.

That's why we're introducing you to Full-Metal Cardio, a crazy-intense, heart-pumping weightlifting regimen that'll get you fitter and leaner than most anything you can do on a $5,000 machine in front of a television. So feel free to sell your treadmill on eBay, and start picking up barbells and dumbbells on cardio day.

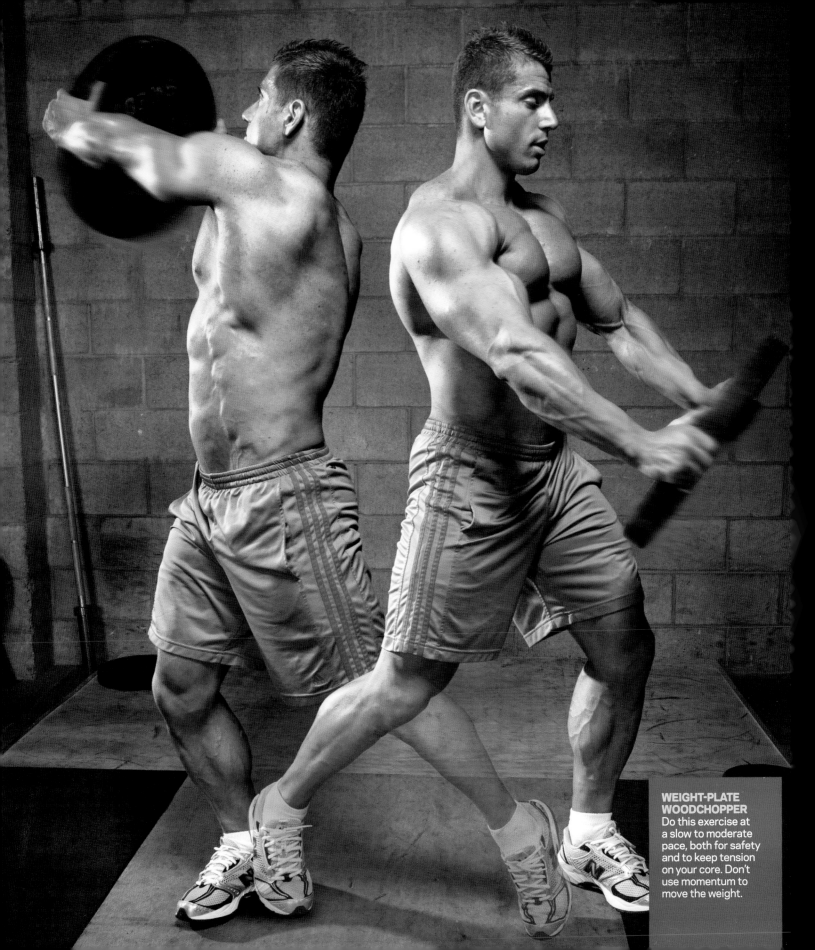

# IRON LUNGS

By now you should be familiar with high-intensity interval training (HIIT), a type of cardio in which you perform short intervals of high-intensity exercise followed by short intervals of low-intensity recovery. For example, on a track, road, or treadmill, you'd alternate sprinting for about 30 seconds with 30–60 seconds of walking until you hit your desired total time. Volumes of research show that HIIT burns more fat than the steady-state variety, even when the steady pace is done for a longer period.

Leave it to us to boost the efficacy—and brutality—of an already effective workout. The following Full-Metal Cardio program uses the same basic premise as HIIT, with one major difference: We're swapping out the treadmill, bike, and elliptical machines for traditional weightlifting exercises that'll hit every muscle fiber in your body to burn more body fat and send your conditioning through the roof.

Besides minimizing treadmill-induced boredom, this program addresses two other main drawbacks of traditional cardio: 1) it's not as effective at burning calories post-workout as weight training is, and 2) most programs work only your lower-body musculature, thus limiting the release of fat-burning enzymes.

Research shows that lifting weights boosts your metabolic rate (calorie-burning) higher and for longer after a workout than cardio does. One reason is that weights provide resistance, which taxes the muscles both biochemically and mechanically. As a result, many calories are expended to return the muscle fibers to their original condition and beyond. Typical cardio provides resistance as your legs propel your body and absorb the landing, but not to the same degree as weight training.

Most cardio—cycling, running, stair-stepping—exhausts the legs while the upper body gets something of an active recovery. Weight training allows you to broaden the scope of muscles you want to involve to include large body parts, such as back, chest, and shoulders. More muscles in need of recovery means more calories being burned to fuel that recovery process over the next several hours or days. Hitting more muscles also turns on more fat-burning enzymes, potentially doubling their activity in your body.

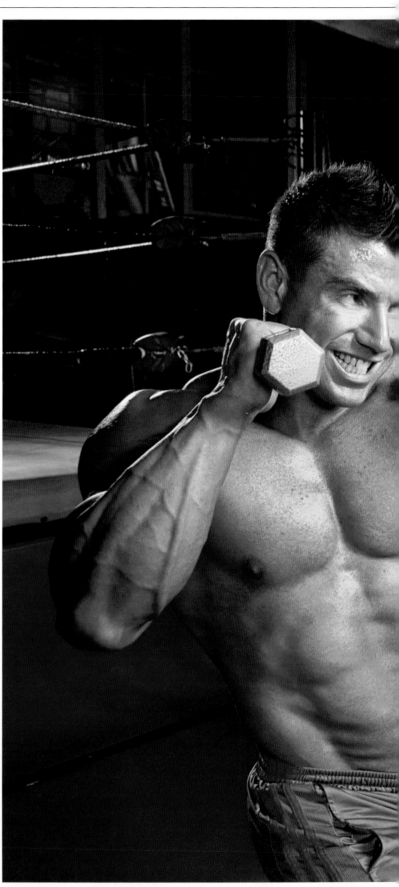

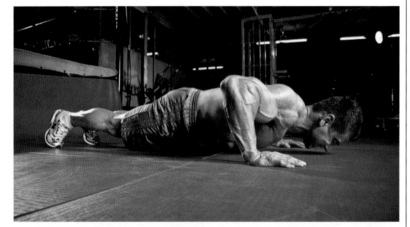

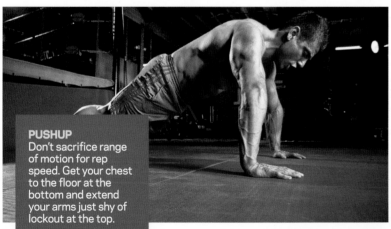

**PUSHUP**
Don't sacrifice range of motion for rep speed. Get your chest to the floor at the bottom and extend your arms just shy of lockout at the top.

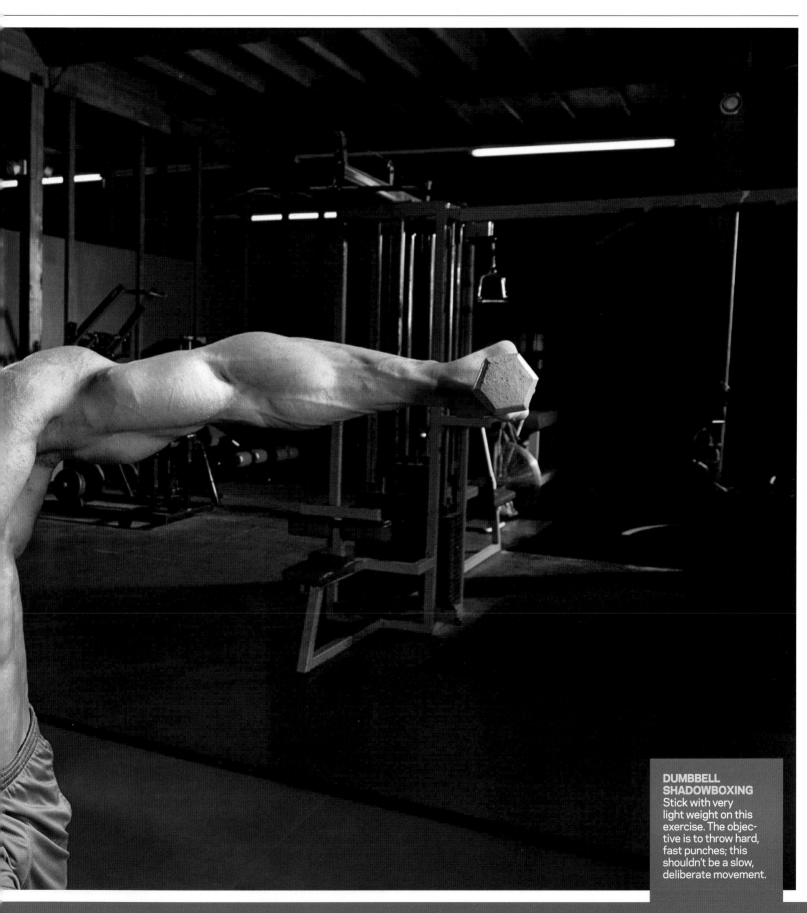

**DUMBBELL SHADOWBOXING** Stick with very light weight on this exercise. The objective is to throw hard, fast punches; this shouldn't be a slow, deliberate movement.

# LIFT TO GET LEAN

Full-Metal Cardio more or less mimics a HIIT scheme: You do one set of an exercise followed by 30 seconds or less of active rest (however long it takes to set up the next exercise), then you do a set of the next move and so on. To promote balance, we suggest you do the same number of exercises for upper and lower body while mixing in full-body lifts such as thrusters and clean and jerks, which are not only great calorie burners but also help improve explosiveness and athleticism. In other words, don't perform solely upper-body exercises in one session, lest you defeat the purpose of maximizing muscle recruitment. The workouts starting on the next page feature the proper balance of movements to get your heart rate up while chiseling away at stubborn blubber.

The training sessions in this program are relatively short, but don't let that fool you—the intensity is such that 10–20 minutes of these circuits is all you'll be able to handle. If it's easy for you, it probably means you rested too long between exercises or didn't go heavy enough on your sets.

We recommend performing one of these workouts one or two times a week on days you don't regularly train—any more than this can easily lead to overtraining and burnout, considering that your muscles will also need time to recover from traditional lifting workouts. To round out your cardio week, feel free to include one or two steady-state sessions. A logical training split might look like the following routine.

Full-Metal Cardio workouts should always be challenging, and progressing within the basic parameters outlined here is very straightforward. Once you can complete a workout in relative comfort, do one or more of the following: Aim to perform more reps in each set, increase weight on one or more exercises for the same number of reps, increase intensity by shortening rest periods between exercises, and/or increase volume by going through the circuit one or two more times. The beauty of HIIT/circuit training is there's no limit to how intensely you can train.

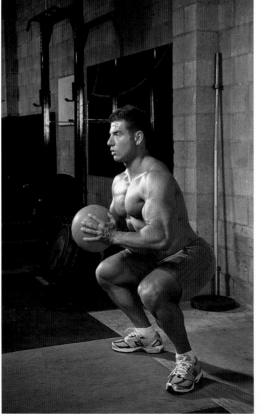
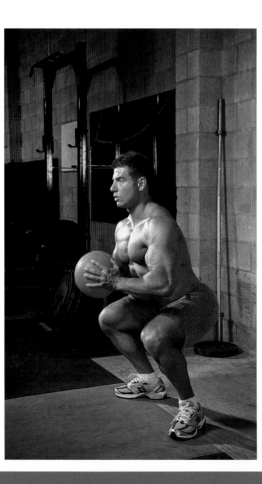
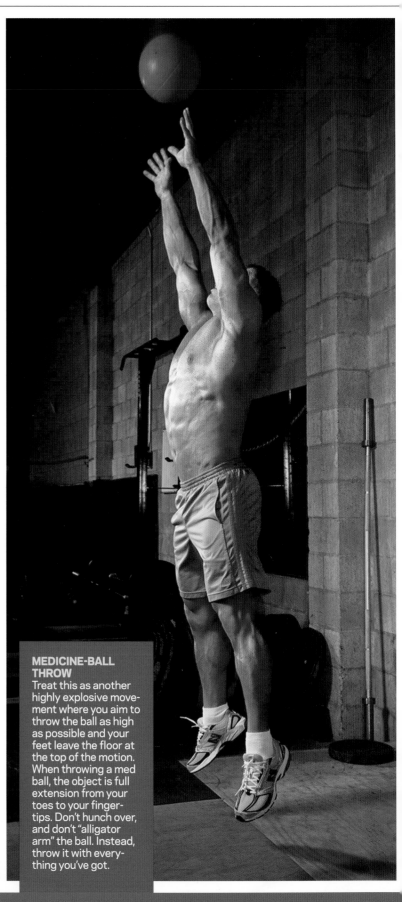

**MEDICINE-BALL THROW**
Treat this as another highly explosive movement where you aim to throw the ball as high as possible and your feet leave the floor at the top of the motion. When throwing a med ball, the object is full extension from your toes to your fingertips. Don't hunch over, and don't "alligator arm" the ball. Instead, throw it with everything you've got.

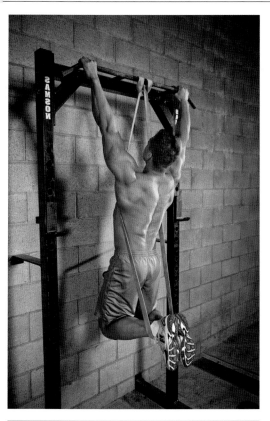

## ROUTINE 1: FIVE-EXERCISE CIRCUIT

| EXERCISE | REPS |
| --- | --- |
| Thruster | 12 |
| Assisted Pullup | 15 |
| Walking Lunge | 10 each leg |
| Pushup | To failure |
| Weight-plate Woodchopper | 15 each side |

*Perform this circuit three to five times with as little rest between exercises as possible. Rest one or two minutes between circuits. The next time you do this workout, aim to shorten your time.*

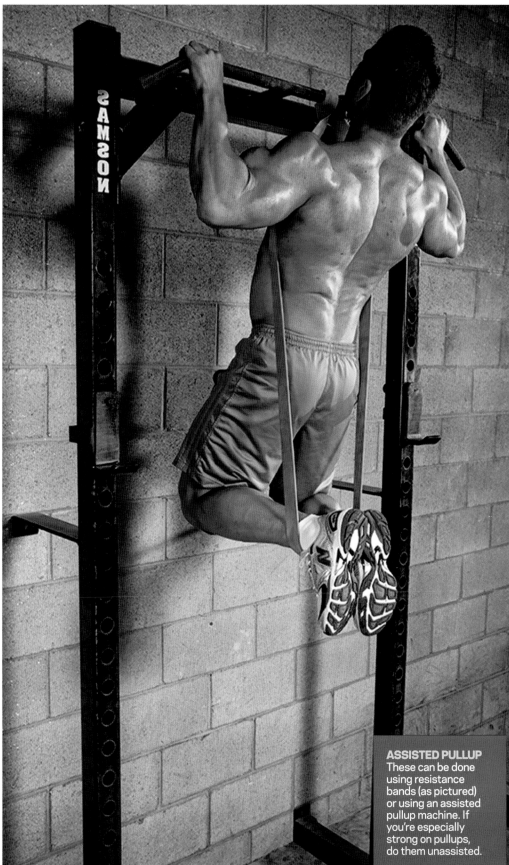

**ASSISTED PULLUP**
These can be done using resistance bands (as pictured) or using an assisted pullup machine. If you're especially strong on pullups, do them unassisted.

## ROUTINE 2: 10-EXERCISE CIRCUIT

| EXERCISE | REPS/TIME |
| --- | --- |
| Jump Squat | 12 |
| Assisted Pullup | 15 |
| Clean and Jerk | 10 |
| Pushup | To failure |
| Dumbbell Swing | 15 |
| Plank | 30 sec. |
| Medicine-Ball Throw | 10 |
| Dumbbell Shadowboxing | 30 sec. |
| Walking Lunge | 10 each leg |
| Jump Rope | 1 min. |

*Perform this circuit three to five times with as little rest between exercises as possible. Rest one or two minutes between circuits. The next time you do this workout, aim to shorten your time.*

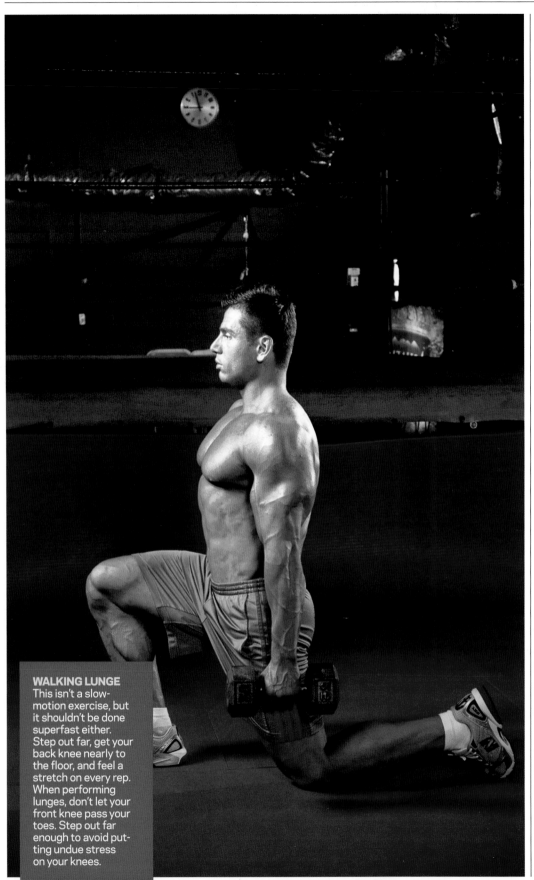

**WALKING LUNGE**
This isn't a slow-motion exercise, but it shouldn't be done superfast either. Step out far, get your back knee nearly to the floor, and feel a stretch on every rep. When performing lunges, don't let your front knee pass your toes. Step out far enough to avoid putting undue stress on your knees.

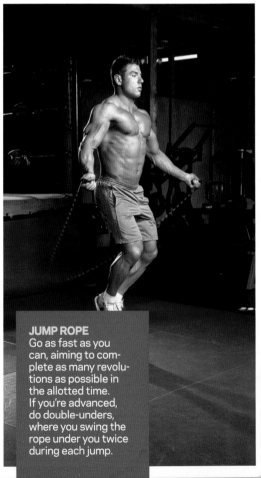

**JUMP ROPE**
Go as fast as you can, aiming to complete as many revolutions as possible in the allotted time. If you're advanced, do double-unders, where you swing the rope under you twice during each jump.

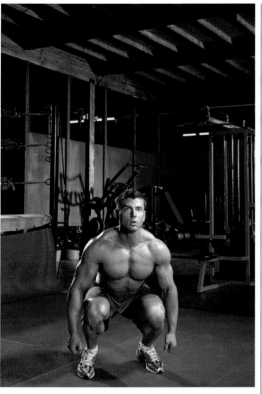

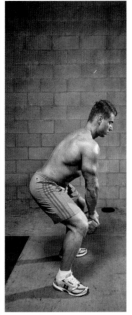

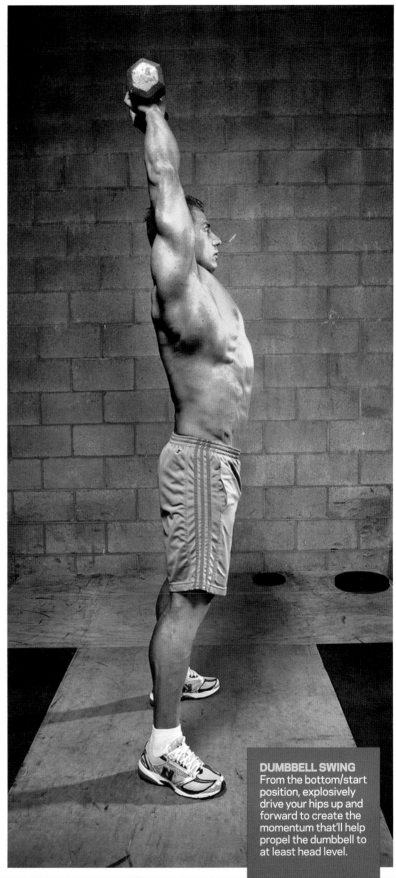

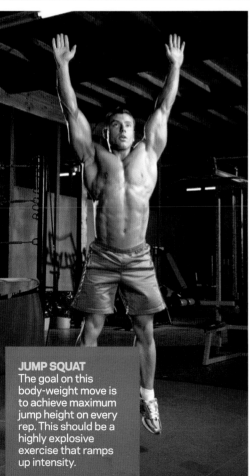

**JUMP SQUAT**
The goal on this body-weight move is to achieve maximum jump height on every rep. This should be a highly explosive exercise that ramps up intensity.

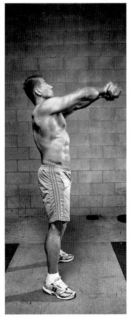

**DUMBBELL SWING**
From the bottom/start position, explosively drive your hips up and forward to create the momentum that'll help propel the dumbbell to at least head level.

## ROUTINE 3: FULL-BODY CIRCUIT
### EXERCISE

**Thruster**

**Dumbbell Swing**

**Clean and Jerk**

**Jump Squat or Medicine-Ball Throw**

**Jump Rope**

*Do each exercise for 30 seconds, performing as many reps as possible in that time. Rest 30 seconds between each exercise. Perform this circuit two or three times, resting one or two minutes between each circuit.*

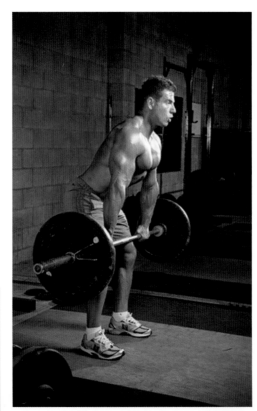

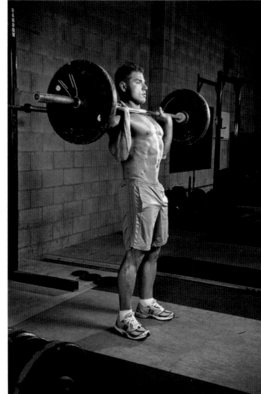

**CLEAN AND JERK**
This is a big, explosive, full-body move with maximum range of motion. When in doubt on weight selection, go light and gradually work your way up.

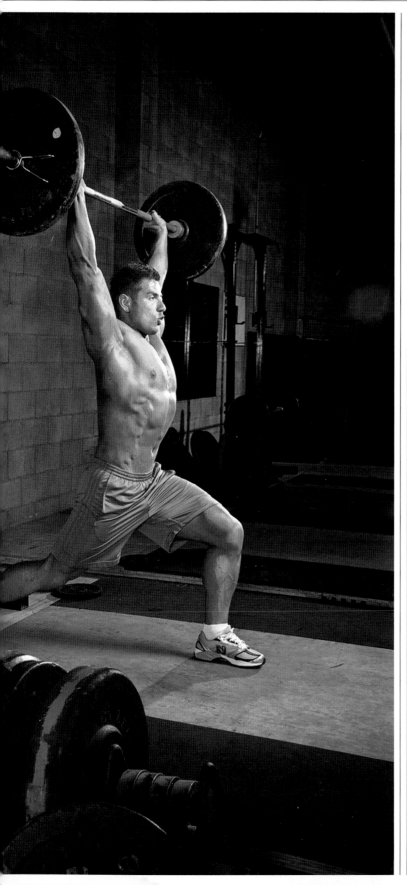

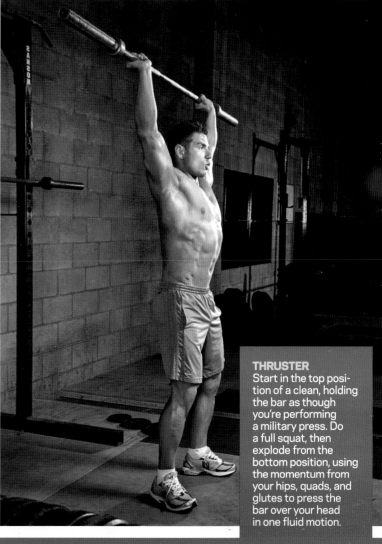

**THRUSTER**
Start in the top position of a clean, holding the bar as though you're performing a military press. Do a full squat, then explode from the bottom position, using the momentum from your hips, quads, and glutes to press the bar over your head in one fluid motion.

# AB EXERCI

*Photographs and/or written descriptions of the following abdominal and*

# SE FINDER

*core exercises can be found on the listed corresponding page(s).*